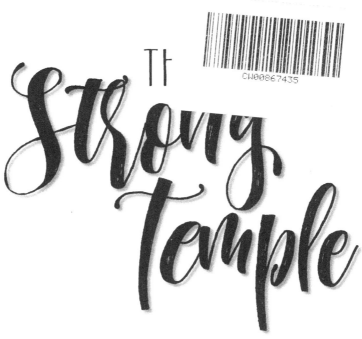

The Strong Temple

A WOMAN'S GUIDE TO DEVELOPING SPIRITUAL AND PHYSICAL HEALTH

Kathryn Baker

with Dr. Wayne Jacobs

Unless otherwise noted, all Scripture quotations are taken from THE HOLY BIBLE, NEW INTERNATIONAL VERSION®. © 1973, 1978, 1984, 2011 by Biblica, Inc.® Used by permission of Zondervan Publishing House. Grand Rapids, Michigan. All rights reserved worldwide.

Scripture quotations marked NLT are taken from the Holy Bible, New Living Translation, copyright © 1996, 2004, 2015 by Tyndale House Foundation. Used by permission of Tyndale House Publishers Inc., Carol Stream, Illinois 60188. All rights reserved.

Scripture quotations marked NASB are taken from the New American Standard Bible®, Copyright © 1960, 1962, 1963, 1968, 1971, 1972, 1973, 1975, 1977, 1995 by The Lockman Foundation. Used by permission. www.lockman.org.

Scripture quotations marked MSG are taken from NIV/The Message Parallel Study Bible. Copyright © 2008. Used by permission of Zondervan Publishing House. Grand Rapids, Michigan. All rights reserved worldwide.

Diagrams and illustrations by M.B. Trogdon. Used by permission.
Editing by Bethany McShurley and ChristianEditingServices.com.
Cover and page design by ChristianEditingServices.com

WestBow Press books may be ordered through booksellers or by contacting:

WestBow Press
A Division of Thomas Nelson & Zondervan
1663 Liberty Drive
Bloomington, IN 47403
www.westbowpress.com
1 (866) 928-1240

Because of the dynamic nature of the Internet, any web addresses or links contained in this book may have changed since publication and may no longer be valid. The views expressed in this work are solely those of the author and do not necessarily reflect the views of the publisher, and the publisher hereby disclaims any responsibility for them.

Any people depicted in stock imagery provided by Getty Images are models, and such images are being used for illustrative purposes only.
Certain stock imagery © Getty Images.

ISBN: 978-1-9736-0269-9 (sc)
ISBN: 978-1-9736-1470-8 (e)

Library of Congress Control Number: 2018910634

Print information available on the last page.

WestBow Press rev. date: 01/30/2019

To my loving and supportive husband,

Stanley, and daughter, Michelle.

God has blessed me with your encouragement,

providing me with new determination

to complete this Bible study.

Love you two!

Do you not know that your bodies are temples of the

Holy Spirit, who is in you, whom you have received

from God? You are not your own; you were bought

at a price. Therefore honor God with your bodies.

— 1 CORINTHIANS 6:19–20

TABLE OF CONTENTS

PREFACE

My interest in writing a Bible study called *The Strong Temple: A Woman's Guide to Developing Spiritual and Physical Health* began with my own story. As a youth I was very active, but I loved to eat! My schoolmates, bless their hearts, loved to call me names like "ugly" and "fat." Over time I learned to exercise more self-control in my nutritional choices, and thankfully I didn't allow a few bad experiences with my peers to sour me on children altogether. Instead, I grew up to combine my passions for nutritional choices, physical activity and spending time with children. I became a physical education teacher and have made physical and spiritual wellness ongoing pursuits throughout my adult life.

Over my thirty years of teaching physical education and coaching, keeping my body in good working order has always been important to me. But when I began to teach at LeTourneau University, I started to wrestle with the Bible's teachings on the value of not just a person's spirit but also a person's body. I learned that a Christian's body is a "temple" for the Lord—a precious gift meant to bring honor to God. Not long after I accepted that truth, I decided to care for my temple God's way. That led to teaching others to do the same.

I have seen *wonderful* things happen as women begin to view their bodies from a biblical perspective and seek to care for them with that viewpoint in mind. I've watched ladies start to love and care for their unique bodies, praying their way into making wise choices—choices that have led to healthful lifestyles, in turn giving them more energy to share God's love and the gospel's light. So positive were the results of these wellness teachings coupled with Scripture, in fact, that a colleague, Dr. Wayne Jacobs, and I began to pen two related resources: the book you hold and a Bible study for men.

The pages ahead include much of what Dr. Jacobs and I have taught over the years. The information is meant to help you, dear reader, better understand God's design for you and to help you systematically achieve and maintain healthful habits for life. We will discuss wellness behaviors, weight management, meal planning, exercise and strength training, stress management, and disease prevention. But this isn't a message about self-improvement. This is a message about allowing God to equip and strengthen you to be your best physical you, for His glory.

Whether you do this study on your own or participate in a group (a leader's guide is included in the back), know that I am praying the Lord will show you how to take care of your precious temple His way.

Blessings of joy!

Kathryn Baker
Adjunct Associate Professor, Kinesiology

ACKNOWLEDGMENTS

As I prepared to send this final copy to the publisher, I was filled with gratitude for my teammate, Dr. Wayne Jacobs. This writing journey was possible only because of his coaching and mentoring. Dr. Jacobs, whom I affectionately call "Dr. J.," is a Kinesiology Professor. His knowledge about wellness and his deep love for God have been so valuable as together we've worked to educate others in healthy living while sharing the life-changing good news about Jesus Christ.

I also extend thanks to LeTourneau University and Mobberly Baptist Church in Longview, Texas. Both entities have provided me with opportunities to teach this material as I worked to develop and refine it. And I cannot mention Mobberly Baptist without saying that I am hugely grateful to my prayer warriors Betty, Kay, and Shirley, to the women's ministry, and to the Bachtell Bible Study Group.

A big thank-you also belongs to Shawna Westervelt for her valuable help with the exercises and stretches and Kelsey Jacobs, who also posed for pictures. And I cannot finish my list of gratitude without mentioning Bethany McShurley of Faith Based Ministry and Karen Burkett and her professional team at Christian Editing Services. Without their patience and guidance, this study would not have made it to print.

God has truly blessed me with these loved ones, encouragers, and friends. Ultimate gratitude belongs to Him. He is so worthy of all glory!

INTRODUCTION

Whether you are a beginner who cringes at the thought of eating healthfully and exercising regularly or are a fitness pro who has adopted wise choices as a lifestyle, you are about to begin a fun journey toward deeper personal wellness and spiritual growth. I wish I could be there to hug your neck and tell you how excited I am to know you have made these topics a priority!

Included in this book are six weeks of personal study content. Each week is broken into five daily sessions that should require only about fifteen minutes to complete—though some of the suggested exercises and worksheets will take a bit longer.

You may choose to complete this book's content on your own or with friends. One of the best parts of this study, in fact, is that it allows you to bring your loved ones, extended family members, prayer warriors, coworkers, and Bible study buddies along! *The Strong Temple* is designed to work as a seven-week group study for those who choose to learn and apply these concepts with others.

To go through this material with a group, simply purchase one book for each participant. Either you or a selected facilitator will use the leader's guide at the back of this resource to enrich the learning experience. The first group get-together is meant to precede the reading of week 1's content. After the first meeting, group sessions will serve to reinforce what participants read throughout the week.

Because of the wellness nature of this study, ten to thirty minutes of mild daily exercise will be encouraged often throughout our time together. For both your personal study time and the optional group sessions, you will need to dress accordingly. (Please complete the Exercise Readiness Questionnaire below before participating in any of the suggested activities.)

EXERCISE READINESS QUESTIONNAIRE (ERQ)

Throughout this study, mild to moderate exercise is encouraged. To ensure that you are ready for exercise, please complete the following.

Yes	No	1) Has a physician ever diagnosed you with a heart condition **and** indicated you should restrict your physical activity?
Yes	No	2) When you perform physical activity, do you feel discomfort in your chest?
Yes	No	3) When you were not engaging in physical activity, have you experienced chest pain in the past month?
Yes	No	4) Do you ever faint or get dizzy and lose your balance?
Yes	No	5) Do you have an injury or orthopedic condition (such as a back, hip, or knee problem) that may worsen from a change in your physical activity?
Yes	No	6) Do you have high blood pressure or a heart condition in which a physician is currently prescribing medication?
		7) Are you pregnant?
Yes	No	8) Do you have insulin-dependent diabetes?
Yes	No	9) Are you 69 years of age or older **and** not used to being very active?
Yes	No	10) Do you know of any other reason you should not exercise or increase your physical activity?

If you answered yes to any of the above questions, talk with your doctor before you become more physically active. Tell your doctor your plan to exercise, and describe the questions you answered with a yes. If you honestly answered no to all questions, you can be reasonably certain you can safely increase your level of physical activity gradually. If your health changes so you might then answer yes to any of the above questions, seek guidance from a physician.[1]

---

1   "Exercise Readiness Testing (ERQ)." Used with permission from *ExRx.net*.

Week One

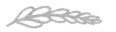

FOUNDATIONS

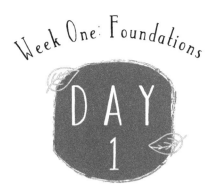

Week One: Foundations

DAY 1

SALVATION'S IMPORTANCE
AND THE ROLE OF THE HOLY SPIRIT

*Please note: If you are completing this study with a group,
read this chapter after your first group session.
If you are reading on your own, dive right in!*

Eat well! Work out. Detoxify! Manage stress. Rest and relax! Article headings like these bombard us in the magazine aisle, in our email inboxes, and during Internet searches. But should these issues have any bearing on the life of a Christ follower, or are they just worldly concerns that pull attention away from what really matters?

What do you think?

_____

_____

_____

As a dedicated Christian and collegiate-level teacher of wellness practices, I've spent a lot of time thinking about this idea. I suggest these concepts do have value for Christian women. In fact, I sincerely believe our interest in them can help us find new fuel for our spiritual journey.

In the pages ahead, I'll discuss physical fitness and general wellness principles in detail, sharing with you about their relevance to day-to-day life. But since the Strong Temple concept around which my thoughts are based rests on a person's spiritual relationship with Christ—a relationship I missed until well into adulthood—I'll spend much of this week on the spiritual foundation underlying our topic.

Head Knowledge

I was raised in a Christian home, went to church regularly, and was surrounded by strong Christians. From the time I was very young, I had "head knowledge" about Jesus. I knew who He is and had a textbook answer for what He came to do. I did not, however, have the heart knowledge that respected Him as Lord and accepted the wisdom of His teachings.

Can you relate? Explain.

_____

_____

_____

_____

_____

_____

_____

Miserable choices characterized many years of my early life. I've come to believe that was because I had only head knowledge of Jesus rather than a relationship with Him. Yes, I did my best to be a good person. But that was mostly because I hoped that being a good girl would be enough to get me into heaven one day. I failed to understand the Bible's teaching that salvation comes from the Lord (Jonah 2:9). I thought earning heaven was all up to me. And so I floundered.

Years of living in spiritual darkness, fear, and unhappiness passed until a season came when I could no longer stand the thought of continuing down my aimless path. After talking to our family pastor and his wife, I finally embraced the importance of salvation in Christ by faith. At last I knew I needed Jesus. I was ready to ask Him into my heart.

Heart Knowledge

I opened my Bible, intent on finding out once and for all exactly what a person must do to gain salvation and the freedom I craved. Jeremiah 31:34 stood out to me. There God said, "I will forgive their wickedness and will remember their sins no more." *Yes!* I thought. *That's what I want!* I desperately desired to be washed clean of my sins. I was more than ready to give my life to Jesus that day as I flipped through Scripture, but somehow I couldn't find the step-by-step instructions. I needed help.

That Saturday morning my husband, who had been a devoted Christian for years while I had only gone through the motions, was *thrilled* when I told him I was ready to accept Christ. He knew just the scriptures I needed to hear. He spoke to me about truths found in the book of 1 Corinthians as well as some in Romans. Then he led me in prayer, asking me to repeat after him and to mean what I said with my whole heart.[1]

---

1   Reciting this prayer was no magical formula for obtaining salvation. Rather, it provided me a tangible way to know I was surrendering my life into God's hands.

19

"Father God," he said, "we come to You today because Kathryn Baker wants to make Jesus Lord of her life. We believe the truth of 1 Corinthians 15:3–4, that 'Christ died for our sins according to the Scriptures, that he was buried, that he was raised on the third day according to the Scriptures.' And we are resting in the truth of Romans 10:9–11: 'If you declare with your mouth, "Jesus is Lord," and believe in your heart that God raised him from the dead, you will be saved.' We are sinners, Lord, who have no hope of heaven except for Your Son, Jesus, who took upon himself the death penalty we deserved. Please forgive us, and help us make choices that honor You from this day forward. In the name of Jesus. Amen."

The prayer ended, and I was so excited. I was overwhelmed with tears of joy! I *felt* Jesus transforming me and washing me clean. I finally knew what *born again* means. I felt the truth of Romans 4:8: "Blessed is the [woman] whose sin the Lord will never count against [her]."

Over the following weeks I read my Bible with focus. I wanted so much to grow in my newfound faith! But a moment of fear hit when I read Philippians 2:12–13: "My dear friends, as you have always obeyed—not only in my presence, but now much more in my absence—continue to work out your salvation with fear and trembling, for it is God who works in you to will and to act in order to fulfill his good purpose." Thankfully, my husband was there to remind me that the verse doesn't suggest that I have to do anything to keep my salvation intact. Rather, it means every Christian needs to commit to making life choices that demonstrate love and gratitude toward Jesus Christ, because God wants to work through us. The best way to honor Him, he assured me, is to keep learning more of Jesus's teachings and to obey them. "God's Holy Spirit will help you," he added.

The Role of the Holy Spirit

I spent a lot of time over the next few years putting my husband's advice into practice. And the more I read the Bible, the more I realized a Christian's life should look very different from that of someone who doesn't know Christ. But I think the moment I stopped feeling intimidated by that idea and began to grow excited at the thought of becoming more like Jesus came when I stumbled across these next verses. They showed me that as a Christian I am literally a temple of God's Holy Spirit, who lives in and works through me!

> Do you not know that you yourselves are God's temple and that God's Spirit lives in you? If anyone destroys God's temple, God will destroy him; for God's temple is sacred, and you are that temple. (1 Corinthians 3:16–17)

> Do you not know that your body is a temple of the Holy Spirit, who is in you, whom you have received from God? You are not your own; you were bought at a price. Therefore honor God with your body. (1 Corinthians 6:19–20)

Since a Christian's body is a temple of the Holy Spirit, Jesus lives in and through us in a sense. Everything we do and the way we treat and use our body are directly related to our relationship with Christ. Once I realized that, I knew I needed to relinquish control and allow the Holy Spirit to lead and guide me. It was time to use my mortal body—my precious temple—to honor Jesus, not because I had to but because I wanted to. Hal-le-lu-yah!

Before we delve further into what I mean, let's pause. Maybe reading my Jesus story led you to question whether you know Him as Lord and Savior. If that's the case, please check out Appendix A at the back of this book. Or perhaps this is the first time you ever thought of your body as a temple of God's Holy Spirit, and you aren't certain what I'm talking about. This diagram may help:

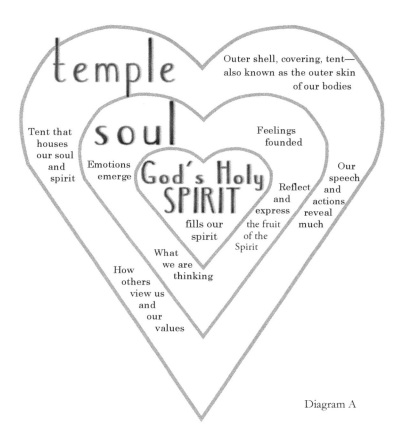

Diagram A

Notice in the illustration that the core of a Christian's being contains God's Holy Spirit. The Greek word for the center of a person's heart is *pneuma*. It means "breath, wind, self, disposition, spiritual state" and can even refer to "the Holy Spirit."[2] Because the breath of an individual is the sign of life, *pneuma* came to mean the "spirit that gives life to the body" as referenced in Scripture.[3]

---

2   Spiros Zodhiates and Warren Patrick Baker, eds., *Hebrew-Greek Key Word Study Bible NIV: New Testament Lexical Aids* (Chattanooga, TN: AMG Publishers, 1996), 1663.

3   Ibid.

The middle heart in the illustration represents a person's soul. "The Greek word *psyche,* with a long *e,* means soul. Specifically, the soul is the seat of the senses, desires, affections, and passions."[4] This is where emotions, will, and feelings are stored. It is from the soul, which should be deeply influenced by the Holy Spirit within it, that a Christian relates to others. Expressions of the fruit of the Spirit—which we will discuss tomorrow—spill out of what is happening within the soul.

The outer heart in the picture depicts the physical body, which is the portion of a Christian that the earlier Bible passages I presented refer to as the "temple" of God's Spirit. The "Greek word *soma* (long *o*) means a material, living human body."[5] The *soma* is like a tent that houses both the soul and the spirit.

As I grew to better understand truths like these during my personal Bible study, I realized that a Christian woman takes the Holy Spirit everywhere she goes. The way she acts, the things she says, even the way she treats her body are reflections of Christ's importance to her. If she is dismissive of His residence in her life, she won't hesitate to disobey God's Word and to treat her body as if it's hers alone. If, however, she respects the Spirit's place in her life, she will seek to honor Jesus through obedience and care of the temple in which He resides. First Corinthians 6:19–20 from *The Message* clarified this for me: "Didn't you realize that your body is a sacred place, the place of the Holy Spirit? Don't you see that you can't live however you please, squandering what God paid such a high price for? The physical part of you is not some piece of property belonging to the spiritual part of you. God owns the whole works. So let people see God in and through your body."

That concept—temple maintenance as a way of honoring a Christian's relationship with the Lord—is the hinge on which this study hangs.

Since the day I met Christ, I've been eager to honor Jesus in all I do and to teach and encourage others to do the same. Let's work together in

---

4   Ibid., 6034–Psyche, 1668.

5   Ibid., 5393–Soma, 1667.

these next weeks to get our temples physically fit! I am so excited you are joining me.

Reflections

What key words or scriptures from today's material do you most wish to remember?

_____

_____

_____

Daily Exercise Prompt

Movement is key to keeping our temples strong and healthy. All you need to get moving is a good pair of walking shoes and some comfortable clothing. If you haven't done so already, please fill out the Exercise Readiness Questionnaire on page 12. Then step outside for a nice, leisurely walk.

You may choose to walk around your home, neighborhood, or workplace for five to ten minutes. If you can, take along a family member, a coworker, or even the dog. Keep a steady pace. While you walk, thank God for your temple and for the promise of heaven—a place where He promises to make our temples new and pain free.

(Bonus points today if you take the time to do a bit of leg-stretching when you finish exercising. Refer to the Stretching Guide, Appendix B, at the back of this book.)

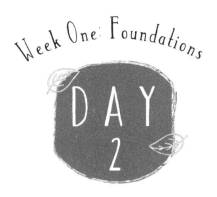

Week One: Foundations

DAY 2

INTRODUCTION TO
THE FRUIT OF THE SPIRIT

When I was a little girl, my godly grandma told me life's journey would be easier if I kept my eyes fixed on Jesus. (She was so right, and I wish I had listened to her back then!) As I reflect on other spiritual conversations we had as she worked to teach me biblical truth, I remember what care Grandma took to help me understand that the Christian life is not all up to me. "Jesus works through His followers, Honey," she'd say. "When we give our hearts to Him and live in obedience, He will produce all kinds of good fruit in our life."

For years I had no idea what she meant, but one day during my Bible study time I came across a passage that explained it. Galatians 5:22–23 lists qualities evidenced in the life of a person who has accepted Jesus as Lord.

Read Galatians 5:22–23 and then list the fruits of the Spirit here:

_____

_____

_____

_____

_____

Once we accept Jesus and set about obeying Him, we are like a branch grafted into God's family tree through Christ. And when that happens, we are positioned to bear all kinds of godly fruit that serve to bless those around us as the Holy Spirit pumps God's love into the fibers of who we are. In fact, love, joy, peace, patience, kindness, goodness, faithfulness, gentleness, and self-control should be character qualities associated with every Christ follower.

Interestingly, this list of godly qualities came from the apostle Paul. Before the world's greatest Christian missionary met Jesus, he was called Saul. And Saul *hated* anything related to Christianity. George A. Buttrick, commentary editor, offers an insightful note on the change this man experienced: "Before [Paul] became a Christian, his sinful nature had been in rebellion against God and at cross-purposes with itself, splitting his life into fragmentary deeds. Then the Spirit came to integrate his life with God and men, centering it in the unifying love of Christ."[6] With this gift of the Holy Spirit, Paul began to notice incredible changes happening in his life. Where once he had hated believers, he began to love them. Where once his heart had felt crippled by jealousy and impatience, he felt peace, kindness, and gentleness. No longer controlled by sin, Paul could exercise self-control. "Each fruit [or character trait] of the Spirit [at work within him]," Buttrick concludes, "was simply love in another form, a revelation of the character of God" at work within Paul's heart.[7]

This same Spirit, *Pneumatos* in Greek, is at work within each modern Christ follower too. And this same fruit, which I will equate with character traits throughout this study, should develop in our life. Building on the illustration we discussed yesterday, the process looks something like this:

_____

6   George A. Buttrick, "Galatians," vol. 10 of *The Interpreter's Bible* (Nashville: Abingdon Press, 1953), 565.
7   Ibid.

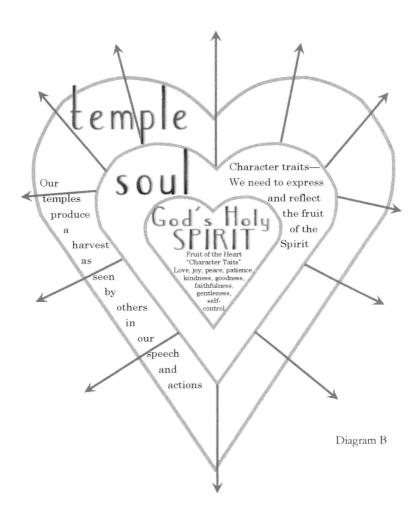

temple

soul

God's Holy SPIRIT

Character traits—
We need to express
and reflect
the fruit
of the
Spirit

Our
temples
produce
a
harvest
as
seen
by
others
in
our
speech
and
actions

Fruit of the Heart
"Character Taits"
Love, joy, peace, patience,
kindness, goodness,
faithfulness,
gentleness,
self-
control

Diagram B

Growing fruit flourishes when its parent branch receives plenty of water. With that in mind, I like to think of the Holy Spirit at work within my heart as a water master who keeps me supplied with what I need to grow in Christlikeness. He fills me with God's love. We will discuss this concept further in a later lesson, but for now let's consider how the Holy Spirit worked in the lives of these Bible characters so we can better understand the importance of His work.

Look up the following to see how the Holy Spirit's activity is described in each of these Bible passages:

Luke 1:41: "Elizabeth was* _____ *with the Holy Spirit."

Luke 1:67: "Zacharias was* _____ *with the Holy Spirit."

Luke 4:1: "Jesus,* _____ *of the Holy Spirit . . ."

Acts 2:4: "[The believers] were* _____ *with the Holy Spirit."

The Holy Spirit's activity is often equated with a *filling*—which brings to my mind the image of water gradually increasing the circumference of a hanging apple. When you and I are filled with the Spirit, we thrive and produce good fruit. However, when we are filled with stress or overbusyness and neglect to spend top-quality time with God through prayer and reading His Word, we tend to wither and bear little fruit.

In the pages to come, I will speak a lot about making time for exercise and healthy eating, and I will turn the character qualities produced by the Spirit into visual aids to help us along the way. Please hear me: Nothing we do for our bodies is as important as spending time with Jesus. Doing so "turns on the faucet" so the Holy Spirit can flow through us and produce things like joy and peace. In fact, we need Him far more than we need to reach fitness goals, because without His love flowing through us by the Spirit's power, nothing we do will have lasting worth.

My pastor recently shared a sermon that has resonated with me as I've prepared this book. He reminded the congregation how often we busy girls (and boys) tend to fill our life with things that don't matter: surfing the Internet, reading pointless books and blogs, taking in hours of sensationalized media, and even trying to reach good goals of little spiritual value. "Put yourself in the position where you can be filled daily with the Holy Spirit," he said. "You can be filled when you stop snacking on the sensational. Then you can feast on the spiritual."[8]

So let's make time to be refreshed by the living water provided by the Holy Spirit. Let's give our relationship with Jesus the time and attention it deserves. As we do that, we will grow in spiritual health and will produce the good things that should be evident in the life of every Christ-follower.

Reflections

What key words or scriptures from today's material do you most hope to remember? Why?

_____

_____

Daily Exercise Prompt

Walk around the outer perimeter of your home or workplace for ten minutes today. If you have an iPod, tune into Christian radio or listen to an audio Bible as you walk. The goal is to spend time with Jesus. Ask Him to let the Holy Spirit fill you and produce good fruit through your life.

After your walk, turn to Appendix B. Stretch your legs with some toe touches and a hurdler's stretch.

---

8   Dr. Glynn Stone, Jr., unpublished sermon series on the Holy Spirit. Mobberly Baptist Church, Longview, TX, September 2014.

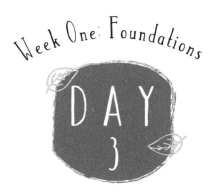

DAY 3

BETTER UNDERSTANDING
OUR IDENTITY IN CHRIST

Over the last two days, we've learned about the Holy Spirit's role in the life of a Christ follower. Yesterday I likened Him to a water master who helps us produce good fruit so others can see Jesus's influence on us. That is my own idea, but it finds its basis in an illustration Jesus used to help His early followers better understand their relationship with God.

Read Christ's words (below) from John 15:1–8. Then in the margin, write out the identities of the vinedresser (the gardener), the vine, and the branches.

"I am the true vine, and my Father is the gardener. He cuts off every branch in me that bears no fruit, while every branch that does bear fruit he prunes so that it will be even more fruitful. You are already clean because of the word I have spoken to you. Remain in me, as I also remain in you. No branch can bear fruit by itself; it must remain in the vine. Neither can you bear fruit unless you remain in me.

"I am the vine; you are the branches. If you remain in me and I in you, you will bear much fruit; apart from me you can do nothing. If you do not remain in me, you are like a branch that is thrown away and withers; such branches are picked up, thrown into the fire and burned. If you remain in me and my words remain in you, ask whatever you wish, and it will be done for you. This is to my Father's glory, that you bear much fruit, showing yourselves to be my disciples."

The following illustration may help solidify this concept in your mind:

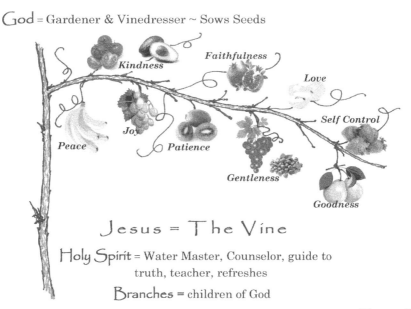

God = Gardener & Vinedresser ~ Sows Seeds

Kindness   Faithfulness   Love

Peace   Joy   Patience   Self Control

Gentleness   Goodness

Jesus = The Vine

Holy Spirit = Water Master, Counselor, guide to truth, teacher, refreshes

Branches = children of God

Diagram C

God, the gardener or vinedresser, freely gave the world His Son, Jesus Christ, as a vine of connection between sinful humans and His own holiness. Those who place their faith in Jesus are grafted into God's family through Him. We Christians become branches who are accepted by God because Jesus has made us holy by dying as a sacrifice for our sin so the Lord remembers it no longer. As branches, we receive nourishment from God the Father and Jesus the Son through the Holy Spirit at work within us. As we allow the work of that water master to flow through our lives and live in obedience to God's commands, we bear spiritual fruit.

In other words, when you asked Jesus into your heart, He became your lifeline, the vine that makes you worthy of God the vinedresser's attentions. As you live in a way that honors God, the Holy Spirit keeps you watered so you will continually grow in Christ-likeness and will develop character traits like peace, love, and self-control. The results of this partnership can be an amazingly sweet harvest that leads others to accept Christ as Lord.

> **How, if at all, does this vineyard imagery change the way you think about your relationship with Jesus?**

_____

_____

_____

> **About the way you think of yourself?**

_____

_____

_____

For me, one of the most helpful aspects of this image is that it reminds me that my relationship with Jesus needs constant tending. It keeps me aware that if I am not growing in Christ, I am missing the whole reason God saved me: He intends for His followers to make a positive difference with their lives. And He makes huge investments in us to see that happen!

Think about it. Vineyards are planted for one reason: to produce sweet, savory grape harvests. Achieving that goal never happens by accident. Vineyards require 24 hours a day and 365 days a year of care by a vinedresser committed to seeing maximum yield.

Importantly, the word *vinedresser* has several meanings, which include "takes away, removes, or even cuts off," but its primary definition is "to lift from the ground."[9] Indeed, the work of caring for grape vineyards is intense. Many vinedressers do all this work by hand. Vines require tucking up between the wires because grapevines left to grow wild will never produce any fruit. Moreover, vines must often be pruned—cut back—to promote ongoing growth.

Day by day, year after year, God is with us, lifting us up, securing us to Him, pruning us toward the kind of spiritual productivity for which He created us: telling others about Jesus, training our children to know God, extending compassion to the poor and helpless, and being all we can be for His glory.

Reflections

What key words or Scriptures from today's material do you most wish to remember?

_____

_____

_____

9   Charles R. Swindoll, *Jesus: The Greatest Life of All* (Nashville: Thomas Nelson, 2007), 92.

Daily Exercise Prompt

Switch things up today by jogging in place for ten minutes. As you do, pray and ask God to produce a sweet, savory harvest through your life. Welcome Him to prune and refine you and to give you a deep desire to please Christ in all you do.

Close your workout time by doing calf and quad stretches as explained in Appendix B.

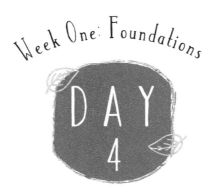

DAY 4

SPIRITUAL FRUIT AND
THE WELLNESS TOPIC

In 2 Corinthians, Paul—yes, the same guy who was formerly called "Saul"—explains something fabulous that happens in our life when we accept Christ and invite His Spirit to work through us. As the Spirit of the Lord works within us, "all of us who have had that veil removed can see and reflect the glory of the Lord. And the Lord—who is the Spirit—makes us more and more like him as we are changed into his glorious image" (2 Corinthians 3:18 NLT).

> *What qualities would you expect to see in the life of someone who is becoming more and more like Jesus?*

_____

_____

_____

Did your answer to that last question include words like *love* and *kindness*, referencing some of the spiritual fruit we discussed earlier? I hope so!

Today we will take a closer look at the fruit of the Spirit by assigning a literal fruit to each of the characteristics Paul said should be evident in the life of a Christ-follower. Doing this will both help us remember what kinds of things we should be producing and will serve as a visual springboard for specific wellness topics I'll cover soon.

> *Think about it. What kind of fruit would you choose to represent love?*_____
>
> *Self-control?* _____
>
> *Kindness?* _____

I've chosen to represent *love* with the **quince apple**. I selected this fruit because God so loved His creations, man and woman, that He placed many fruit trees in the garden to provide nourishment for them. As several classical paintings show Eve eating an apple, the link is easy for me to remember. *Forbearance*, or *patience*, is represented by the **kiwi**. I selected this because it takes patience to peel one of those sweet green fruits! *Goodness* is represented by the **pear**. I like this link because it depicts a typical shape of a healthy woman. *Kindness* is represented by the **avocado** and the **tomato**. I like the **avocado** as a visual representation because it contains healthy oils and fat that feed the heart. **Tomatoes** were chosen because they have four chambers, as do our physical hearts. *Joy* is represented by **green grapes**; they are a blood-vitalizing food that feeds muscles. *Gentleness* is represented by **red grapes** and **blueberries**. Both fruits contain antioxidant agents that help fight cancer cells. I picked **strawberries** to depict *self-control*, to restrain from over-indulging. *Peace* is represented by **bananas**. I like this association because this fruit gives us quick energy to combat stress. I also eat bananas to give my temple potassium to discourage muscle cramping when sleeping. And finally, *faithfulness* is represented by the **pomegranate**. I chose this fruit because to me it represents the seeds of truth that God plants in our heart as we read His Word. This helps us to be faithful to abide in Him.

On the visual below, I've placed inside a horn of plenty—or a cornucopia--the representative fruits I chose. This type of container is typically displayed around Thanksgiving and is "filled with an abundance of the earth's harvest."[10] I like this image, because it reminds me to give thanks for the good and abundant spiritual fruit the Spirit wants to produces through us.

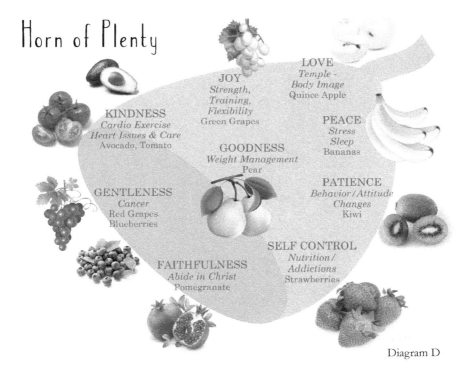

Diagram D

Although the visual links made between grocery store produce and spiritual fruit here are my own, I want to emphasize that the fruits of the Spirit are *literal* traits meant to be applied in actual situations. God's power at work within us, for instance, produces love so we might love on others through encouraging words and good deeds. It produces gentleness to help us respond to difficult people with a soothing approach rather than hostility.

---

10   "Cornucopia," *Society for the Confluence of Festivals in India: http://www.thanksgiving-day.org/cornucopia.html* (July 12, 2016).

You may have noticed, however, that alongside the spiritual fruits listed on the visual aid I included some unusual terminology—most of which you may expect to find in a health and wellness study. These applications are purely figurative. I've chosen to use them with the goal of better anchoring our later discussions in the Word of God. We will look at the reasons more closely in the weeks ahead.

Reflections

What key words or scriptures from today's material do you most wish to remember?

_____

_____

_____

_____

Daily Exercise Prompt

Take a look at the horn of plenty diagram, and select the spiritual fruit that seems most lacking in your life. As you walk briskly around your home or workplace for ten minutes today, ask the Lord to produce that specific fruit in you. Think about ways you have seen that fruit show up in the lives of others. When you are finished, do the calf and quad stretches listed in Appendix B.

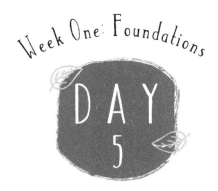

Week One: Foundations

DAY 5

WELLNESS EXERCISE BASICS

Now that we've laid the spiritual basics behind this study and you've—I hope—grown accustomed to getting up and moving at the close of each daily lesson, let's shift gears. Today I want to address several terms that will prepare you for the upcoming weeks of growing emphasis on physical activity.

First, understand that as sure as I care about your spiritual condition and thus emphasize activities like Bible reading and prayer, I am also concerned about the health of your physical heart and body. For that reason, I want to help you see the need for cardio exercise. The word *cardio* refers to the heart, arteries, and other blood vessels that carry blood through our temple to sustain life. These cooperative parts are known as the cardiovascular system, which enables us to carry out even the most basic activities at home, work, school, or while at play.

Cardio Fitness

Cardiorespiratory (or aerobic) exercise increases the ability of our heart and lungs to transport oxygen through cells and tissues to our muscles. Such exercise supports the ability of our temple to maintain a flow of oxygen. It strengthens the circulatory system, which carries nutrients to the body and removes carbon dioxide. The strength of this system, in fact, helps us sustain prolonged physical exercise.

Performing cardio fitness or aerobic activities requires some serious oxygen intake! In fact, anytime you work out for more than two minutes, you engage in aerobic activity that will require you to draw in additional oxygen to continue that activity. Working at regular activities like sweeping and vacuuming, as well as performing motions like swimming and cycling, can help get the heart rate up so the body will more efficiently pump oxygen through the organs and into extremities. Over time, this builds physical endurance.

Cardiorespiratory exercise contributes to achieving a healthy Body Adiposity Index (BAI), which I will discuss later. It is also quite helpful in reaching and maintaining a healthy body weight. Many who exercise this way regularly insist it contributes to a good night's rest. (I'd call that a bonus!)

Strength Training

Strength training, a preferred term in this study, is a common way of referring to resistance training or weight training. This type of activity, which sometimes involves lifting weights, helps us build muscle tone and gain strength. Over time it will improve the strength of our heart and will allow us to perform daily tasks with ease. Lunges, squats, Pilates, PiYo, and push-ups are simple strength-training that can be performed in the comfort of our home. Following a regular strength-training regimen may even contribute to improved mental cognition and stress reduction.

Changing the Mind-Set

Many people encounter exercise terms like these and cringe at the thought of exercising regularly, but getting off the couch or out of the office chair and asking our bodies to move is so good for us! A healthy goal, in fact, is doing thirty minutes of cardio exercising three to five days each week as is discussed further in week 4's content. This should be supplemented with the kind of basic strength training we will discuss in week 5.

If the very thought of starting such a routine causes hives, know that making such a change—if indeed an exercise routine would require a change for you—is not something that happens overnight. Rather, getting there is best accomplished through small steps. And think about it: for the past four days, assuming you participated, you have been up and working at exercise for at least ten minutes a day this week. (Congratulations to you!)

Let's set some simple goals that will lower any anxiety you may feel about exercising.

In the list below, circle at least three wellness goals that sound doable. These will help you in the process of making daily exercise a priority.

- I will exercise one day a week for a month.

- At my desk I will set a timer to remind myself to get up and move at least once an hour for a duration of at least two minutes.

- I will walk at least three times a week, slowly working up to that goal.

- I will ask family members or friends to exercise with me.

- I will join a local gym to help me get started in attaining better fitness

- I will go to yard sales to buy some inexpensive workout equipment and will use it.

- I will look for sales where I can purchase a good pair of walking shoes.

- I will purchase a Fitbit or a heart monitor.

Now, in the following list cross out the sentences that best reflect any negativity you may have toward working out and healthy living.

- I don't like any form of exercise.

- I don't like to get sweaty.

- I don't have time for exercise.

- Losing all this weight would take forever.

- My temple is not built for working out.

- No one will exercise with me.

- I'm too embarrassed to work out in public.

- It is too expensive to purchase workout equipment or join a gym.

- I like my unhealthy snack foods and sodas.

- I am unwilling to lower my risks for diseases by changing my poor eating and exercise habits to create a healthier lifestyle for myself.

By responding to those last activities, you identified simple personal goals toward wellness and symbolically shut down your own reservations about making fitness changes. Now let's gauge just how much (or how little) you may need to do to make the kind of health adjustments I'll discuss in the following chapters. Please candidly respond to the following:

Wellness Survey

Read the following questions, marking an X on the right side of the question if you can answer yes or an X on the left side of the question if you answer no.

NO   **YES**

1   Do you exercise regularly?

2   Do you refrain from smoking and using smokeless tobacco products?

3   Do you eat well-balanced meals and healthy snacks?

4   Do you maintain your recommended body weight?

5   Do you get seven to eight hours of sleep most nights?

6   Do you use stress management techniques?

7   Do you consume alcohol in moderation or avoid it altogether?

8   Do you use medication as prescribed and only when needed?

9   Do you surround yourself with healthy relationships?

10   Do you wear a seatbelt and observe the speed limit?

The number of *X*s on the right side of the continuum represent the good choices you make toward your wellness. Each *X* on the left side represents an area where change could help you improve your general wellness.

If we are honest, most of us had a few *X*s on the left side of our continuums. And if you have more than a few, don't berate yourself. Picking up this study shows your willingness to improve, and that is half the battle. Your first goal, regardless of your answers above, is to recognize the power of making wise choices.[11] I hope that by the end of this study, regular exercise and smart food selections will be among the wise choices you make.

Reflections

What do you most wish to remember about today's content?

_____

_____

_____

_____

Daily Exercise Prompt

Today let's get very practical about exercising. Vacuum the whole house, take the dog or baby for a walk, or go for a bike ride. Whatever you choose to do, set the goal of moving constantly for ten minutes today. Get that heart pumping in a cardio workout that doesn't match what normally comes to mind when people think of getting fit. Don't forget to do a bit of stretching when you finish. Look at Appendix B if you'd like help.

---

11   Wayne Jacobs, with Kathryn Baker, _The Strong Temple: A Man's Guide to Developing Spiritual and Physical Health._ (Bloomington, TN: Westbow Press, 2015), 6–7.

Week Two

CATCHING THE VISION

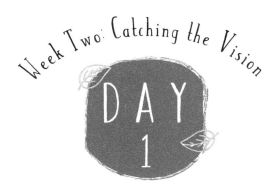

SPIRITUAL AND PHYSICAL WELLNESS

Spiritual Wellness

Wellness is all about being fit and confident. But before focusing on physical wellness, let's consider what *spiritual* wellness involves. (Remember, physical wellness is of little lasting value without it.)

As I shared last week, my life was long characterized by poor choices and general uneasiness. But when I received Jesus as my Savior, I became a new creation who lives with the assurance that heaven is waiting for me at the end of my earthly journey. This gives me a sense of fullness, direction, and purpose. I believe this is the truth at the heart of what Jesus meant when He said, "I have come that they may have life, and have it to the full" (John 10:10). Because of my relationship with Christ, I can confidently go to God in prayer and trust the advice I find in His Word for everything from building a long-lasting marriage to getting along with difficult people. I can know that my personal value to God is immense. He is the center of who I am and what I do, and that brings me such joy!

Having spiritual wellness—which the Bible teaches is achieved only through a relationship with Jesus—really changes how a person thinks about self in relation to God and others. When we know Jesus the vine, we have a positive view of ourselves as beloved children of the Creator. What we look like ceases to matter so much. And as we get to know Him better, we begin to think of others as either sisters and brothers in Christ or as individuals who need to know the love of their heavenly Father. Comparing ourselves with others or worrying over what they think about us takes a backseat to encouraging them along their own life journey.

We are declared spiritually well at the moment of salvation, but engaging in activities that honor our relationship with Jesus is an important part of *knowing* that we are spiritually fit. Such things are like getting off the sofa to go for a walk or running as a reminder that we can do so; they inform us about the true fitness of our souls.

Place a check mark beside each activity you believe would foster a person's sense of spiritual wellness.

_____ Reading the Bible daily

_____ Giving to support the church and missions work

_____ Obeying God's Word

_____ Attending church regularly

_____ Praying continually

_____ Serving the poor

_____ Participating in Bible study

_____ Telling others the good news about Jesus's death and resurrection

All the above activities support Christian growth and keep us mindful of our spiritual wellness. Making them a regular part of your life will contribute to your overall sense of well-being.

Physical Wellness

Physical wellness is "good physical fitness and confidence in [one's own] personal ability to take care of health problems."[1] It is associated with having good cardiovascular health, muscular strength, and flexibility. Those who desire to be physically well are often the same people who eat healthful foods, get regular exercise, manage their stress, and get enough rest. They also make healthy decisions like avoiding the use of excessive alcohol or harmful drugs or the misuse of prescribed medications. These people have medical check-ups and screenings regularly. Their decisions are geared toward extending quality of life into the golden years.

Many people think of physical wellness in terms of how a person looks. They equate it with bodybuilders who have muscles galore or with fitness gurus who work out every time the gym door is open. But wellness doesn't look like a muscle man or a swimsuit model. (Thank goodness!) Wellness is more about achieving the energy and tone necessary to walk, lift, push, pull, and bend our way through daily activities. It is about having the mobility to move about freely with ease and without pain throughout our lifetime.

In their book *Christian Paths to Health and Wellness*, writers Peter Walters and John Byl note that exercise and being physically fit "can help you have a strong heart, [an] enhanced immune system, [help you reach your] recommended body weight, lean body mass, healthy body fat index, [and can contribute to] improved nightly rest, management of stress in your daily

---

1   Werner W. K. and Sharon Hoeger, *Lifetime Physical Fitness and Wellness: A Personalized Program* (Belmont, CA: Thomson Wadsworth, 2007), 11.

life, [and] improved cognition. . . . It can help to prevent and or delay the risk of diseases."[2]

Which of the following words best describes your current level of wellness?

Poor

Lacking

Average

Good

Terrific

Up to now, what have you done to pursue physical wellness?

_____

_____

What benefit of wellness most appeals to you? Why?

_____

_____

I sincerely desire that each Christ follower live in a temple that is both spiritually and physically fit. Whether you are just beginning your journey to the kinds of wellness discussed today or are seeking to mature further, remember that every step you take to strengthen your relationship with Jesus or to foster

---

2   Peter Walters and John Byl, *Christian Paths to Health and Wellness* (Champaign, IL: Human Kinetics, 2013), 79–84.

the health of your body is one taken in the right direction. Make the time to celebrate the positive changes you've made so far.

Reflections

What key words or scriptures from today's material most appealed to you?

_____

_____

_____

Daily Exercise Prompt

Grab your bicycle and helmet for a quick ride, your tennis shoes for a power walk, or go for a brief swim. The goal today is to get your heart pumping with fifteen minutes of cardiovascular exercise. When you are finished, do two or three of the stretches found in Appendix B.

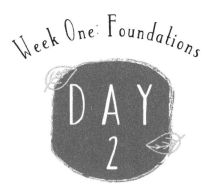

Week One: Foundations

DAY 2

RESPONDING TO THE IMAGE IN THE MIRROR

Love is one of my favorite spiritual fruits or character traits. We first saw it in our introduction to the Spirit's work in the life of a Christian. I selected the quince apple to represent it. The Greek word for *love* in reference to the Spirit is *agape*. According to one commentary, "Agape love shows kindness and self-sacrifice regardless of whether the object of the love is worthy or even likeable."[3] And that is why I have chosen to link love with today's topic.

Friends, you need to love the lady who greets you in the mirror each morning, even if you've been telling yourself "you aren't worthy" or "nobody likes you" lies for years. Whether or not you think she deserves your kindness and dedication, the woman in your mirror is incredibly valuable to God. You must learn to see and value yourself the way He does.

---

3 Thoralf Gilbrant, ed., *The Complete Biblical Library: New Testament Study Bible* (Springfield, MO: The Complete Biblical Library,
   1986), 225.

In the last group session you were asked to take a good long look in the mirror. If you haven't done so already, grab a hand mirror and answer these questions:

How do you view yourself physically?

_____

_____

_____

What do you think God sees when He looks at you?

_____

_____

_____

We live in a culture that constantly screams, "Your hair isn't right! Your clothes are out of date! You need to diet! You need to get in shape! Your teeth need to be whitened! Your face could use a good lift!" Unfortunately, we've grown so accustomed to the constant bombardment of marketing ploys like these that we've started to believe them. Many of us look in the mirror and see only "flaws." And we assume that everyone else, including the Lord, also sees us as a poor project in need of complete overhaul.

It is time to work on our biblical view of self. Throughout the Bible God states His unconditional love for us, His precious daughters. Followers of Jesus are of all shapes and sizes and hair types and ages—and are beautiful and worthy in His sight.

Look up the following scriptures and match them to the insights they reveal about your value to God:

1. _____ Jeremiah 1:5

A) God sent Jesus to die for me even when I was a sinner.

2. _____ Psalm 139:13–14

B) God formed me and knew me even before I was in the womb. He set me apart.

3. _____ Matthew 10:30

C) God ordained my days.

4. _____ Romans 5:8

D) God made me "fearfully" and "wonderfully." As His work, I am wonderful.

5. _____ Psalm 139:16

E) God knows how many hairs are on my head. He misses no detail about me.

The correct answers are B, D, E, A, and C. The book of Genesis explains that God made humanity, both male and female, in His own image and then pronounced them "very good" (Genesis 1:27–31). Each of us is a treasured gift shaped by the hands of our heavenly Father. We are, in all our differences, priceless works of art who are cherished by the Master Designer.

If fact, I like to think of people as designer's originals. Consider this: Just as no two snowflakes are alike yet each is beautiful in its own way, individuals are unique and special. Even identical twins are delightfully different—just another indication of God's endless creativity and love for humanity.

Sarah E. DeWeerdt of the *Genome News Network* sheds light on the way the Creator's design works. Our uniqueness comes down to our genomes. She states,

> A genome is all of a living thing's genetic material. It is the entire set of hereditary instructions for building, running, and maintaining an organism, and passing life on to the next generation. . . . In most living things, the genome is made of a chemical called DNA. The genome contains genes, which are packaged in chromosomes and affect specific characteristics of the organism.[4]

> Genome variations are differences in the sequence of DNA from one person to the next. Just as you can look at two people and tell that they are different, you could, with the proper chemicals and laboratory equipment, look at the genomes of two people and tell that they are different, too. In fact, people are unique in large part because their genomes are unique. . . . Every human genome is different because of mutations—"mistakes" that occur occasionally in a DNA sequence.[5]

What Sarah DeWeerdt calls "mistakes" are the tweaks to our genetic coding that God makes to give humans fabulous variations in eye and hair color, build and bone structure, fingerprints, and many others. They are little foundation stones deep within our precious temples that make us individuals, and the biblical truth is that there's no "mistake" to it. Each of us is divinely created and so cherished by the Father. He loves us so much that He sent His Son, Jesus, to die and return to life so we may spend forever with Him if we will only believe He did this to forgive us of our wrongs and to make us clean.

Over the years as I have taught the concepts presented here, I've marveled at the way God can use this simple message to help women see themselves through the lens of His love and grace. Below are the testimonies of three

---

4   Sarah E. DeWeerdt, "What's a Genome?" Posted January 15, 2003. *Genome News Network*: *http://www.genomenewsnetwork.org/resources/whats_a_genome/Chp1_1_1.shtml#genome1* (July 19, 2016).

5   Sarah E. DeWeerdt, "Genome Variations," posted January 15, 2003. *Genome News Network*: *http://www.genomenewsnetwork.org/resources/whats_a_genome/Chp4_1.shtml* (July 16, 2016).

students who now view themselves as designer's originals and are enjoying the blessings of doing so.

> "It has taken me a long time to reach the point of maturation where I can honestly say, 'I believe that I do love myself!' . . . I have learned to love myself because I am exactly who God made me to be: me!" *(AR)*

> "God created me, and no matter the shape I possess, I still love me. . . . The Lord . . . created me for a specific purpose and a specific design. No matter the curves, I believe God can still use me, and God still loves me. I want to show God's love through me to everyone around me. God gave me my smile to be infectious, and God knew what He was doing. I LOVE ME!" *(RH)*

> "I . . . love the Lord with all my heart and therefore enjoy the fact that He gave me a sense of humor, creativity, and my height of five-feet-two inches tall! My short stature has helped me to be more accepted into this community [where my family is doing mission work]. God's plan for me to be here began before I was born! Jeremiah 1:5a says, 'Before I formed you in the womb I knew you.'" *(IBS)*

Friend, I so desire—and the Lord Jesus so desires—that you will embrace that woman in the mirror as a beloved treasure who was created with care and designed with purpose.

As we close today, read through the list below to guage how well you love your temple. Place a check mark beside all that apply. The more boxes you mark, the more agape love you are extending to yourself.

_____ I engage in positive self-talk.

_____ I read my Bible daily.

_____ I take care with daily grooming.

_____ I share scripture with my Bible study buddies or fellow
          prayer warriors.

_____ I pray for my family, friends, and the world.

_____ I am growing daily in my relationship with the Lord.

_____ I share the gospel with those to whom the Holy Spirit
          directs me.

_____ I smile to reflect God's love.

_____ I put healthy foods into my temple.

_____ I exercise my temple often during the week.

_____ I try to get at least eight hours of sleep a night.

_____ I refuse to look at airbrushed images as points of comparison.

_____ I manage my stress in healthy ways.

Reflections

What key words or scriptures from today's material do you most wish to remember?

_____

_____

_____

_____

Daily Exercise Prompt

Get your blood moving with fifteen minutes of the activity of your choice. Then complete your workout by doing some of the stretches listed in Appendix B. Remember—exercising is one way to show love and care for yourself. You are God's amazing creation!

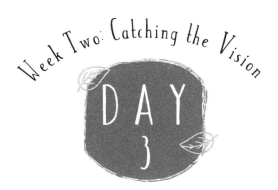

Week Two: Catching the Vision

DAY 3

SETTING GOALS FOR
MY STRONG TEMPLE

The character trait or spiritual fruit of focus today is patience, which I like to associate with the kiwi. The Greek word for *patience* as used in Galatians 5:22 is **makrothumia.** This term means "to be long-suffering [or to have] forbearance . . . [and to utilize] self-restraint before proceeding to action."[6] According to *Webster's New Ideal Dictionary,* long-suffering is equated with "long and patient endurance of offense."[7] In today's lesson we will take precise body measurements before considering what fitness goals we should set for the weeks ahead. The work we will do is challenging, and the goal setting can feel intimidating. I ask for your patience as we walk through this lengthy day of content together. It may help to remember that "patience is . . . a . . . supernatural outcome of being filled with the Holy Spirit."[8]

---

6   Spiros Zodhiates and Warren Patrick Baker., eds., *Hebrew-Greek Key Word Study Bible NIV.* New Testament Lexical Aids.   (Chattanooga, TN: AMG Publishers, 1996), 939.

7   *Webster's New Ideal Dictionary* (Springfield, MA: G. & C. Merriam Company Publishers, 1978).

8   Beth Moore, *Living Beyond Yourself: Exploring the Fruit of the Spirit* (Nashville: LifeWay Press, 2007), 119.

Below we will fill out what I like to refer to as our strong temple stylish information. Knowing the numbers requested will help you keep track of how healthy you are now and can become in time. These numbers will give you a starting place to maintain or improve your temple's shape and wellness. To begin, **please write today's date here:** _____. That will give you a solid baseline should you choose to repeat this exercise and check your progress later.

The first number you'll need is your blood pressure. To get that, you may use a home blood pressure cuff, visit the pressure machine at your local drugstore, or visit your doctor's office. Normal blood pressure, the rate at which the heart muscle is contracting and relaxing, is 120 over 80. Optimal pressure is 115 over 75. **What is your current blood pressure?** _____ (We will discuss the importance of this measurement in a later chapter.)

The next number needed is your BMI number, which will inform you whether you are underweight, normal weight, overweight, or obese. This number also will help you determine if you are at risk for diseases, especially heart problems and diabetes. In this next section, I am drawing from *The Strong Temple: A Man's Guide to Developing Spiritual and Physical Health*, a resource I co-authored with Dr. Wayne Jacobs, to walk you through how to find your BMI:

> **Determine your Body Mass Index by consulting a BMI scale online: http://www.bmi-calculator.net/. Once you've brought this address up on your computer, follow these steps:**

1. Write your weight in pounds: _____

2. Write your height in feet and inches: _____

3. Type the numbers into the BMI scale. (Alternate scales can be found online.)

4   Record here your BMI number as well as any additional insights you have gained about it:[9]

_____

_____

_____

Getting the next set of numbers you'll need will require the use of a soft sewing tape, which can be purchased at any craft store should you not have one handy. Next week we will use these numbers to determine BAI, and they can serve as a good base line as you work to attain or maintain a healthy shape. But for today, let's just take the measurements.

Use a tape to determine the circumference of the following parts, writing your answers in inches below:

Neck   _____

Chest   _____

Wrist   _____

Waist   _____

Hips   _____

Thighs   _____

Calves   _____

This last set of numbers may require you to schedule a visit with your primary care physician if you've not done so lately. *It will require blood work.* **As soon as possible, fill in the following:**

---

9   Wayne Jacobs with Kathryn Baker, *The Strong Temple: A Man's Guide to Developing Spiritual and Physical Health.* (Bloomington, IN: Westbow Press, 2015), 67–68.

Cholesterol Total _____

Cholesterol is a waxy substance existing in two types and is found in animal fats (lipids) and oil. A healthy total is less than 200 mg.

HDL _____

HDL is the **healthy** type of cholesterol, which helps remove fats from the body and prevents plaque from forming in the arteries. A normal HDL number is 40–60 mg or below.

LDL _____

LDL is the **lethal** type, and it tends to release cholesterol into the arteries. This causes many health issues. The optimal or low-risk score for LDL is 100–129 mg.

Triglycerides _____

Triglycerides circulate most of the fat in our diets through our blood. In combination with LDL, they speed up the formation of plaque in our arteries. Less than 150 mg is desirable.

In day 5 of week 1 I asked you to fill in the Wellness Survey. Flip back to that activity, and select one to two areas that you could work on in an effort to improve your physical health. Write those below in statement form:

1. _____

_____

_____

2. _____

_____

_____

Collecting all the above information serves an important purpose. It helps us evaluate ourselves fairly so we may gain a better idea of what areas need improvement. It also allows us some insight into what kinds of changes we need to make to become more physically fit and healthy. For instance, Polly's BMI may reveal that she needs to gain a great deal of weight, and her responses to the Wellness Survey may suggest that smoking and a lack of stress management could be contributing to her weight issue. If that is the case, Polly should consider tackling all three matters at once to ensure best results.

Few overcome the kind of hurdles we are discussing today without first crafting a careful plan for doing so. That's why I encourage you to set goals that can help you along the path to wellness. In fact, it is wise to set STRONG goals leading to your desired destination. *STRONG* is an acronym that leads to effective goal-setting and goal-keeping. *S* stands for specific; *T* is for time-sensitive; *R* is for reverent; *O* is for obtainable; *N* stands for necessary; and *G* means that attaining goals should be guided by those who will hold you accountable. The following example shows how STRONG works.

Let's say my BMI information (or perhaps a recent conversation with my doctor) reveals that I need to lose six to eight pounds as soon as possible. My Wellness Survey reminded me that I rarely eat healthful foods or exercise. I know I need to make changes to correct these issues, but I need to do so through small, easily attainable steps. Losing six to eight pounds within thirty days without making corrective measures to get there would prove pointless.

The STRONG *S* step reminds me I need specific and measurable goals to reach my end goal of losing weight. I also need to make course corrections in other related matters. Therefore, my *S* step might look like this:

To facilitate my weight loss, I will add leafy green vegetables to two out of three meals daily.

I will replace my daily sodas with water. (The research of Peter Walters and John Byl indicates that the best way to consume water is to drink half your body weight in ounces daily.)[10]

I will exercise five days a week, thirty minutes a day.

Once my goals are set, I must make sure they are time sensitive, as the T step reminds me. That means they need to start and end at set times. Moreover, they should include some type of a reward for me to increase my motivation: perhaps I'll shop for a new outfit or pair of shoes, treat myself to a meal at my favorite restaurant, join a gym, or indulge in a hobby if I reach a certain milestone. My *T* step, then, might look like this:

I will add leafy green vegetables to two out of three meals daily for the next thirty days. On day thirty-one, I can buy those new shoes I've been wanting.

I will gradually replace my daily sodas with water until I am drinking water for one full month. On the first day of the next month, I will reward myself with a Dr. Pepper.

I will exercise five days a week from 6:00 to 6:30 a.m. for thirty days. On day thirty-one, I will take a day off to sleep during my usual workout time.

The *R* step reminds me that efforts to reach fitness goals must be reverent— that is, respectful—toward the Lord and toward my body. Reaching goals should not interfere with my pursuit of spiritual disciplines like Bible reading and prayer. They also shouldn't be so aggressive that I cannot attain them without injury—physical or emotional. When I keep these things in mind, my *R* step might look like this:

I will move my morning devotion time to the evening to pursue my fitness goals. I will check inches lost every other week, refusing to be discouraged and remaining quick to congratulate myself.

---

10   Walters and Byl, *Christian Paths*, 175.

Week 2 / Day 3

Step *O* is not entirely unlike step *R.* Goals must be obtainable. It makes no sense to create goals for myself unless they are reachable, and that may occasionally require that I extend myself grace. My *O* step might look like this:

If I miss a day of leafy greens, proper fluid intake, or exercise, I will not punish myself. I will just get back on track the next day.

Step *N* is all about making sure the things I've decided to do are necessary, not superfluous. Making too many changes at once or pushing too hard to reach a target weight in little time will only set me up for failure. Thus, my *N* step—a step designed to double-check the do-ability of my plan—might look like this:

If I want to lose weight, eating greens, trading sodas for water, and getting exercise are important. Yes, following through on my plan will require change, but it is necessary. And it will not hurt me.

And finally, step *G* for guided experience requires that I enlist help or accountability in reaching my goals. Proverbs 13:20 cautions us always to have wise counsel surrounding us. Making changes like those we are discussing will go far more easily if I seek guidance from those who love me and will pray for me as they routinely gauge my progress. My *G* step might look like this:

I will ask Anne and Gena to pray with me over this matter of trying to lose six to eight pounds in thirty days. I will ask each of them to text me once a week to make sure I'm sticking to the plan.

Some find that step *G* is **the** key to success. For that reason, pause to fill in the requested information below so you can begin thinking about your personal support sisters. The women in your home, at your job, in your church, or even those in your Strong Temple study group are all good accountability candidates.

My picks for accountability partners include . . .

1. _____

   Her number is _____

2. _____

   Her number is _____

3. _____

   Her number is _____

Now, scan your answers to the strong temple stylish information and the Wellness Survey question covered above. Then create two to three goals for achieving success in your problem wellness area(s) by using the acronym STRONG. See my examples if you get stuck.

Specific:

_____

_____

_____

Time Sensitive:

_____

_____

_____

Reverent:

_____

_____

_____

Obtainable:

_____

_____

_____

Necessary:

_____

_____

_____

Guided Experience:

_____

_____

_____

Reflections

What do you most wish to remember about today's lesson?

_____

_____

_____

Daily Exercise Prompt

Today do the cardio activity of your choice. Complete your workout by doing stretches listed in Appendix B.

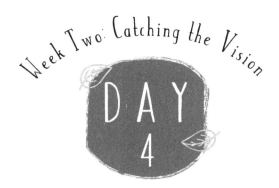

DAY 4

A LOOK AT WHAT KINDS OF THINGS NEED TO CHANGE AND WHY

Yesterday we used the acronym **STRONG** to create personal fitness goals. (I do hope you found it helpful. This method has proved a huge blessing to me!) Today's lesson is about altering our attitudes and sinful behaviors so things like complaining or being lazy won't stand between us and success. As sure as a butterfly pecks through its cocoon and into the glorious freedom of flight, you too can break out of the old habits and behaviors that hold you captive to less-than-ideal health. It all comes down to heart change, to trading sinful tendencies for better choices.

In her Bible study entitled *Jonah: Navigating a Life Interrupted*, author **Priscilla Shirer provided this formula:**

Behavioral Change – Heart Change = Temporary Change

Heart Change + Behavior Change = Permanent Change[11]

---

11   Priscilla Shirer, *Jonah: Navigating a Life Interrupted.* (Nashville: LifeWay Press, 2010), 65.

In other words, if we say we want to change our behaviors but don't make any course corrections within our heart, any change we make will be temporary at best. For instance, Lois might say she's going to give up sweet iced tea and goes without it during fall and winter. But unless something changes deep down in her heart, she's going to pick that sweet tea back up when warm weather rolls around. Drinking iced tea in the sunshine is a long-time habit that makes her feel good. Without a mentality change, she won't go without it for long. If, however, she takes her doctor's diagnosis of diabetes to heart and realizes that unhealthy sweet tea will work on her system like a poison, she will go without it permanently. She'll realize the folly of selfishly indulging in something that could harm her.

In 2 Corinthians 5:17 the apostle Paul said, "If anyone is in Christ, the new creation has come: The old has gone, the new is here!" This passage reminds us that once we belong to Christ, we don't have to be slaves to the things that controlled us before we met Him. Sinful habits like gossiping, overeating, or indulging in lustful thoughts or selfishness can be overcome. The key is to see our hang-ups for what they are: sinful tendencies that can—like a diabetic's sweet tea addiction—hurt us.

Consider the fitness goals you made yesterday. Which sins might you need to overcome to meet your goals? Underline your responses.

> *Indulging pride*
>
> *Gluttony*
>
> *Slothfulness*
>
> *Complaining*
>
> *Jealousy*
>
> *Selfishness*
>
> *Drunkenness*
>
> *Other:*

All the above sinful tendencies can lead us into behaviors that can not only derail our plans to get fit but also injure our relationships with others. Acknowledging the lingering presence of such behaviors in our life is an important step toward getting rid of them. Confessing our mistakes to God is just as important, for as 1 John 1:9 says, "If we confess our sins, he is faithful and just and will forgive us our sins and purify us from all unrighteousness." Jesus wants us to repent of our past mistakes and sins so we will not be held captive to shame and guilt. Once we have repented, we can move on to changing our attitude(s) and behavior(s). It takes self-restraint and patience to make these changes.

> **What specific attitudes and behaviors will you need to change to meet your fitness goals?**

_____

_____

_____

Answers to that last question will vary widely, but we need to refrain from any action that conflicts with meeting our fitness goals—whether that is reaching for the salty snacks or complaining when we must rise earlier than usual to get in shape. It helps to remember we make wise changes not just for self or even for our families. The wise choices we make honor our relationship with the Lord. Remember, our body is His temple.

Consider this passage from Romans 12:1–2 (MSG):

> Here's what I want you to do, God helping you: Take your everyday, ordinary life—your sleeping, eating, going-to-work, and walking-around life—and place it before God as an offering. Embracing what God does for you is the best thing you can do for him. Don't become so well-adjusted to your culture that you

fit into it without even thinking. Instead, fix your attention on God. You'll be changed from the inside out. . . . God brings the best out of you.

As surely as He spiritually matures us when we make the effort to read our Bible regularly, pray, and seek to obey Him, the Lord is faithful to walk beside us as we ask His help in terminating sinful behaviors and attitudes that can sideline our efforts at wellness. With this in mind, I like to hang on to this passage from Deuteronomy 31:8: "The LORD himself goes before you; he will never leave you nor forsake you. Do not be afraid; do not be discouraged."

If you're like me, you've read today's content with the awareness that there are indeed things you need to change. And that can feel overwhelming! But take heart. You don't have to do anything on your own. God will help you if you will just ask and believe He can.

Before we wrap up today, I want to introduce a tool that helps me when I realize that I need to make adjustments. You will find the "Strong Temple Attitude and Behavioral Change Contract" on the following page. ***Please fill it out and keep it in mind as you work toward healthy choices and a positive outlook.***

The Strong Temple Attitude and Behavioral Change Contract

Sum up your attitude or behavioral challenges in one sentence.

_____

How will hanging on to these issues hinder you from reaching your fitness goals?

_____

Who can help you overcome these challenges?

_____

In the list below, select two techniques you can use this week to help modify your attitude and behaviors.

___ Praying regularly to God, your help

___ Deciding to get up and take small steps to accomplish a needed change

___ Finding times to plan wise choices that counter poor habits

___ Reminding yourself of the consequences of continuing on your current path

___ Reading your Bible daily, using a commentary to look up passages about perseverance

___ Attending a church where the Bible is taught faithfully

___ Sticking to a daily routine

___ Getting educated about or seeking Christian counseling on the issue(s) you battle

___ Putting yourself in an environment that will encourage gratitude and positive growth

___ Enlisting a person or group of people to talk to and pray with

Fill in the following based on your answers above:

As of _____ [today's date], I vow to stop

_____ so I may honor my relationship

with Christ and aid myself in reaching my fitness goals. To make this change, I

will _____

and _____.

Signed, _____ [your name].

Reflections

What do you most wish to remember about today's lesson content or the verses within it?

_____

_____

_____

Daily Exercise Prompt

Today do the cardio activity of your choice. What about a good jog or a thorough dusting of the whole house? Complete your workout by doing stretches listed in Appendix B.

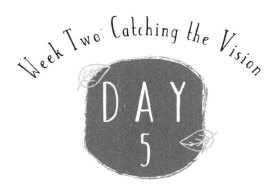

Week Two: Catching the Vision

DAY 5

LEARNING WHERE TO TURN FOR HELP

In a culture all too ready to bombard us with advice, we cannot be too careful in choosing which voices are worthy of our attention. The most important book of wisdom in a Christian's life is, without doubt, the Bible. Our most valuable resource after that is the Holy Spirit, our water master, at work within us. Trusted Christ followers who honestly seek to honor Him in all they do can also be a source of help—that's why I so stress accountability throughout this study. But today I'd like to suggest that you and I as disciples of Jesus have constant access to an additional source that can help us to choose wisely. I will call it self-discipline.

What I mean is that you and I have what we need to get the job done, whether we are trying to be intentional about spending more time in God's Word or losing weight. Each day we are confronted with opportunities to choose in favor of changes that need to be made or to make decisions that run counter to our goals. Ultimately our success or failure in reaching personal goals is traced to whether we remained disciplined in our choices.

Read that last sentence again. Tell about a time when self-discipline helped you reach a personal goal.

_____

_____

_____

_____

One change I've made that has helped me remain disciplined in the pursuit of my goals involves writing vision statements. These are essentially just brief action plans that help me remember where I want to be in the not-so-distant future. I write them as prayers to keep me mindful of the fact that the Lord is my constant help. By keeping copies of these statements in places where I see them throughout the day, I give myself constant reminders to stay on track in making choices that support my vision.

In a moment we will look at vision statements regarding fitness. But before that, I want you to see two examples of how this simple tool can be applied in both spiritual and marriage matters.

The following vision statement reflects this woman's desire to allow her relationship with Jesus to shape who she is:

> Lord, I wish to serve You, my Savior, with an open, willing, and joyful heart. I pray that all whom I encounter will feel the peace and joy that belongs to a child of God. I pray to reflect boldly God's light, love, and gospel truth with those who are hurting and lost, with widows, and with orphans. May my actions reflect You! Please help me to pray daily for myself, my husband, my family, my friends, my church, and the world.

This one shows a missionary's determination to stay the course:

> Lord, today I am serving You through evangelism to Bedouin women, and I am training others to share the gospel. I know You are calling me back to the environment of Human Resources. Please help me continue to make a positive impact for You through faith and transparency.

This one shows a woman's determination to make her marriage a priority:

> God, please enable me to be a Proverbs 31:10–31 wife daily! Show me how to be a "Smokin' Hot Mama" to my husband, offering him the same passion I see in the Song of Solomon. Help me live in a fit temple so I may do all this more effectively. May I encourage and support him as I help complete the purposes you have designed for him. Lord, help me pray for my husband to be the man You wish him to become.

Now let's shift gears. The following examples are vision statements written with specific *wellness* goals in mind. Notice that they too are written as prayers.

> Abba, Father, I willingly surrender my temple to You to use as You see fit. May I continue to care for and love this precious gift. I will care for it physically by what I think and say to and about others. I will exercise on a regular basis. I will endeavor to consume water daily, eat healthier foods, and limit my sweets. I will endeavor to get plenty of rest and manage stressors.

> God, You have made me in Your image. In thanks, I want to live a healthy and disease-free life. Please help me do this. Help me live a life of joy in which I give thanks for all things.

There is no specific formula for writing a vision statement. Just think about the fitness goals and behavioral or attitude changes you've decided to make this week, and consider how God might receive glory should you follow through with them. What improvements would you see in your life? Ask the Holy Spirit to guide you, and **write your vision statement below. Two to five sentences would be good.**

My Strong Temple Vision Statement:

_____

_____

_____

_____

_____

In the weeks ahead I hope you will refer to this statement often as you seek to remain disciplined in reaching the goals you've set.

As we close out this week, let me leave you with a favorite verse that I think ties in beautifully with today's subject: "Whatever you do, work at it with all your heart as working for the Lord. . . . It is the Lord Christ you are serving" (Colossians 3:23–24).

Reflections

What do you most wish to remember about today's lesson content or the verses within it?

_____

_____

_____

_____

Daily Exercise Prompt

Today walk around your home or workplace at a steady pace for fifteen minutes. If bad weather gets in your way, pop in a workout DVD like Leslie Sansone's Christian-based "Walk the Walk, Firm Walk." You may also choose to create your own exercise routine using the ideas included on page 122 in week 4 Day 2. Don't forget to stretch those warm muscles after your workout!

Week Three

NUTRITION AND
WEIGHT MANAGEMENT

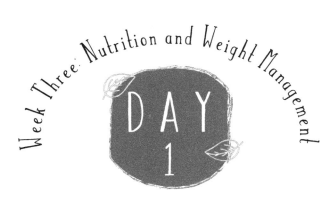

Week Three: Nutrition and Weight Management

DAY 1

FOOD AS NOURISHMENT

If you are doing this study on your own, you may enjoy completing the worksheets "God's Creation of Food" and "God's Pharmacy" before proceeding. They may be found on pages 216 and 217.

As we discuss nourishment this week, I want to begin by considering the spiritual fruit or character trait of goodness. "The Greek word for *goodness* is *agathosune*. . . . It refers to the 'kind actions of individuals.'"[1] I chose the pear to represent this concept, because it reminds me of the natural curves of the average woman's body. Friend, we need to extend goodness—kind actions—to ourselves when it comes to thinking about our bodies and making wise choices about how we will fuel them.

---

1   Thoralf Gilbrant, ed. *The Complete Biblical Library: New Testament Study Bible.* (Springfield, MO: The Complete Biblical Library, 1986), 28.

Our culture often presents consuming food as a form of entertainment and self-indulgence. But if we are to understand food as the source of nourishment it is intended to be, we must learn to view it from a biblical perspective.

Food is first mentioned in the book of Genesis when the Lord notes He was giving people and animals every green plant to eat. In the week prior to making that statement, God had created soil and sun and everything else needed to sustain human life. Everything He made was "very good" before human sin entered the picture.

When Adam and Eve disobeyed God, the curse of sin quickly led some animals to begin consuming each other. We know this because by Noah's day, the earth "was corrupt and . . . filled with violence," and God's wrath against it was aimed at not only His human creations but also the animals (Genesis 6:11–20).

When Noah stepped off the ark, God allowed humans to begin consuming meat as well as plants (see Genesis 9:3). While this might at first seem an odd concession, we must remember that the perfect creation Adam and Eve enjoyed at time's beginning was annihilated in the flood. Environmental changes no doubt made many of the usual foods relatively scarce for some time.

We must not think that because in the beginning humans were vegetarians, abstaining from meat is a secret to wellness. In 1 Timothy, Paul reminds us that since the Lord has approved the consumption of all kinds of food, we should accept them with gratitude: "Food—perfectly good food God created to be eaten heartily and with thanksgiving by Christians! Everything God created is good, and to be received with thanks. Nothing is to be sneered at and thrown out. God's Word and our prayers make every item in creation holy" (1 Timothy 4:2–5 MSG).

Another passage that supports this idea is 1 Corinthians 10:31: "Whether you eat or drink or whatever you do, do it all for the glory of God." In both instances,

Paul was instructing the Christians to eat what they needed to have energy, using even their meals as opportunities to do life for the glory of God.

What most stands out to you about this biblical view of food?

_____

_____

_____

Veggies and meats, fruits and nuts, salty snacks and savory ones were all created by God for our consumption. If we eat them with thanksgiving, we do well. But a word of caution. In a society where many of us can afford to eat as much as we want as often as we like, gluttony—overeating—is a real concern. If we consume more food than we need, no matter how healthful those foods are or how gratefully we receive them, we will set ourselves up for health problems ranging from obesity to gout to just plain not feeling well.

Six Basic Nutrients

One of the best modern tools we have for avoiding over-indulgence and for using food as God intended is an understanding of how food works and what different foods are designed to do.

For starters, we must grasp that our bodies break down food into calories. Calories, according to *Merriam-Webster's Collegiate Dictionary*, are "unit[s] of heat and energy producing value in food when oxidized in the body."[2] Most women need anywhere from 1,600 to 2,000 calories a day.

---

2   *Merriam-Webster's Collegiate Dictionary*, 10th ed. (Springfield, MA: Merriam-Webster, Incorporated, 1993), 163.

It's easy to approximate how many calories we are consuming per meal by taking a quick look at the nutritional information provided on the packaging of our groceries. To achieve weight loss, we need to consume fewer calories. To gain weight, we need to consume more calories than our temple can burn in a day.

Within the calories we ingest are six basic nutrients: carbohydrates (carbs), lipids (fats), proteins, vitamins, minerals, and water. In the following paragraphs, I am adapting material from the book *Christian Paths to Health and Wellness*, by Peter Walters and John Byl, to explain how these nutrients work and where they are typically found.[3]

Carbohydrates, provide short term energy to our temple. They fuel the body and brain. Some good carbs, like those found in sprouted grain bread, whole grain pastas, whole oats, brown rice, spelt, millet, quinoa, sweet potatoes, and dark green veggies, burn fat and release their sugars slowly into our system. These raise our HDL levels. (Yay!) Bad carbs, found in white foods like rice and pasta, break down sugars quickly and thus contribute to our LDL levels. Nutritionists suggest that 45 to 65 percent of an individual's daily diet should be comprised of healthy complex carbs.

Protein has the power to promote physical growth and repair and to provide a major source of energy. It helps build new tissues, antibodies, enzymes, and hormones. Meat, eggs, and dairy products are all good sources of this nutrient. Our temples need between 10 and 35 percent of our daily calories to come in the form of protein.

Lipids or **fats** provide long-term energy as well as insulation and protection for our temples. While lipids need to be consumed in moderation, they are a vital part of the human diet. They are the most energy-rich nutrient, helping to transport vitamins A, D, E, and K throughout our systems. They also help conduct nerve impulses and cushion vital organs. Fat serves as a

---

3   Peter Walters and John Byl, *Christian Paths to Health and Wellness.* (Champaign, IL: Human Kinetics, 2013), 162–75.

thermal regulator and makes up a large portion of bone marrow as well as brain tissue.

Importantly, there are several different types of fats—all of which are typically understood to make food taste better. Saturated fats, which get a bad rap because they are thought to raise cholesterol levels, come from processed meats, animal fat, lard, whole milk, cream, butter, cheese, ice cream, and hydrogenated oils. Unsaturated fat can be found in olive oil, canola oil, and peanut oil. Polyunsaturated and monounsaturated fats tend to lower cholesterol. These are found in corn oil, cottonseed oil, walnuts, sunflower seeds, and soybeans. It is suggested that 20 to 35 percent of our caloric daily intake comes from mainly healthy fats.

Vitamins—found in fresh fruits and veggies—are essential organic substances used by the body for metabolism, protection, and development. Vitamins are critical for blood coagulation and the production of energy, hormones, enzymes, and antibodies. While vitamins are needed only in small doses, they are still vital to proper body function. Without them, our temples can have serious health deficiencies. Talk to your doctor to find out if you need supplemental vitamins.

Minerals help build our bones and teeth. They aid in muscle function and the nervous system's activity. They help maintain the body's delicate acid balances, regulate muscular and nervous tissue impulses, blood clotting, and normal heart rhythm and aid in the production of both hormones and enzymes. Minerals exist in milk, yogurt, cheese, leafy green vegetables, salmon, healthy nuts, whole grains, eggs, enriched grains, soybeans, legumes, and bananas.

Water, which I feel is the most important nutrient for many reasons, is essential to the proper overall function of our temples since our bodies consist of 50–70 percent water. Although it does not contain calories, water aids many bodily functions. For example, it dissolves and carries the nutrients for the body as well as removes waste. It helps regulate the body's temperature and does so much more. While bottled water has gained popularity in recent years, filtered tap water can provide exactly what we need. Consuming eight eight-ounce glasses of this liquid remains a wise nutritional goal. Still, consult with your doctor about what is the best quantity considering your weight and health history.

Reflections

What do you most wish to remember about today's lesson?

_____

_____

_____

Daily Exercise Prompt

Go to the nearest exercise equipment store, and park near the back of the lot so you'll take some extra steps on the way to the door. Once inside, purchase a jump rope. Make sure its length is correct for your height. Step on the middle of the rope—the handles should come just up to your armpits. (Most ropes will allow you to adjust the length by shortening or lengthening the rope at the handles.) When you get home, jump rope for two minutes with your new fitness aid, and thank God for the wonderful foods He provides for us. Don't forget to stretch when you are finished, especially your legs.

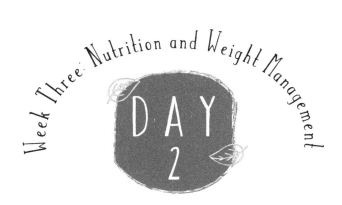

Week Three: Nutrition and Weight Management

DAY 2

UNDERSTANDING THE DIGESTIVE SYSTEM AND TAKING THE CONFUSION OUT OF MEASUREMENTS

Digestive System

Before we begin an in-depth discussion about weights and measurements and why they matter, let's pause to appreciate the amazing digestive system God created within us to process the foods He provides. I love the Lord made such an efficient design for a critical system of our body. He is so very good!

The digestive system begins in the mouth, where our teeth tear food into small particles and saliva helps to break it down. Once food and drink are swallowed, the digestive process becomes involuntary. The esophagus, the long tube between the mouth and gut, squeezes the food until it reaches the stomach. There it sits for about an hour after a meal while stomach acids further digest it. After that, the processed food travels into the small intestine, where most nutrient absorption occurs. According to *Christian Paths to Health and Wellness*, this narrow, twisting tube is about twenty feet long; it fills most of the lower abdomen.[4]

---

4   Ibid.

About three to six hours after meal consumption, the same source explains, food and digestive juices pass into the large intestine. This organ is about five feet long. Over the course of twelve to fourteen hours, it performs several important functions: it absorbs water and dissolves salts; it provides bacteria to promote the breakdown of undigested materials; and it moves leftover matter toward the rectum, where it is stored until elimination.[5]

Taking the Confusion Out of Measurements

The process I've just outlined tells the story of how food travels through our bodies. We have not yet discussed what happens when too little food is consumed or when so much is ingested that the body has far more than it needs. When we fail to take in enough calories, our bodies lose essential fat and may even face organ damage—not to mention that we can end up looking emaciated. Should we take in too many calories, our bodies begin to store the extra as fat. Either of those problems often advertises itself in unhealthy results on body mass.

The remainder of this day's content will revolve around using height and weight and other standard measurements to get a better sense of whether we are consuming what we need or should make adjustments.

First, let's take a closer look at our Body Mass Index, or BMI. Last week in day 3 you figured your BMI number using an online calculator. If you've ever wondered why your doctor begins every office visit by having you step on the scale while a nurse measures your height, it's to attain this number. (I gain weight and shrink in height just thinking about the process!) Doctors use the BMI to figure out whether you are at a healthy weight for your height and to gain insight into whether you are at a risk for illness.

Although it's an okay tool, the BMI alone is not the most accurate measurement, particularly when used on those with a high muscle mass

---

5   Ibid.

gained through strength training. Muscle is denser than fat. Thus, stepping on a scale and calculating our health via a simple BMI does not reveal the full story. This is why I prefer to know my Body Adiposity Index (BAI), which is a more precise number. This figure is a calculation of the percentage of our body fat compared with the rest of our body. It measures lean body mass. It helps us grasp what our bones, muscles, and organs weigh.

To compute your Body Adiposity Index (BAI), grab that soft measuring tape we used last week, and visit this website: **http://www.shapesense. com/fitness-exercise/calculators/body-adiposity-index-calculator. aspx.**[6]

Record your BAI here: _____

Let's say Susan's BAI is 24.4 percent. If you look at the chart provided at the bottom of this same web page, you'll see that Susan, at age thirty-six, is within the healthy range of fat. Moreover, if about 25 percent of her body weight is fat, that means any additional weight revealed on the bathroom scale is a measurement of the base weight of her organs and frame.

The base weight is not something we should alter. As you probably noticed on the website chart, we ladies need a portion of our bodies to be fat because that is how we are designed. This brings us to our next calculation. How can we know what our ideal body weight should be to help us gain a more accurate understanding of what changes we may need to make?

1   Record your current weight: _____

2   Record your BAI, current percentage of body fat: _____

3   Record your desired percentage of fat (between 21 and 38 percent is recommended for most women):[7] _____

6   "Body Adiposity Index Calculator." Posted 2016. "Shape Sense Fitness Exercise Calculators." *Shape Sense.com*: *http://www.shapesense.com/fitness-exercise/calculators/body-adiposity-index-calculator. aspx* (July 26, 2016).

7   Female athletes in serious training, like those preparing for the Olympics, usually have a much lower percentage of body fat than those of us who exercise according to the American Heart Association's standard recommendations.

4. Multiply your current body weight (#1) by your current body fat percentage (#2) to find the weight of your fat: _____

5. Subtract your fat weight (#4) from your body weight (#1) to determine your lean body mass, your weight without the fat: _____

6. Determine your recommended body weight using this formula: Divide your weight without fat (#5) by this calculation: 1.0 minus the desired percentage in #3. (Don't forget your decimal in front of the percentage number before subtracting): _____

For example, a 200-pound female with 30 percent body fat desires to get down to 25-percent body fat. The equations would look like this:

200 lbs. x .30 = 60 lbs.

200 lbs. – 60 lbs. = 140 lbs.

Recommended body weight would equal 140 lbs. divided by (1.0 - 0.25) = 187 lbs.[8]

Now that we've taken the mystery out of the importance of these measurements, let's get practical.

Flip back to your STRONG goals. What, if any, changes might you need to make to your goals based on the information you've gathered here?

_____

_____

_____

8   Wayne Jacobs with Kathryn Baker, *The Strong Temple: A Man's Guide to Developing Spiritual and Physical Health.* (Bloomington, IN: Westbow Press, 2015), page #.

Now let's use our findings to determine the number of calories you *need* daily.

Multiply your recommended body weight (RBW) by your activity level. Use RBW x 13 if you are sedentary; RBW x 14 if you are moderately active; and RBW x 15 if you are active.

Approximate your needed daily caloric intake: _____

Reflections

What did you find most helpful about today's lesson?

_____

_____

_____

_____

Daily Exercise Prompt

Go for a fifteen-minute walk, or spend some quality time with your new jump rope. Do a bit of stretching when you finish exercising. Try to incorporate at least one new idea from Appendix B today.

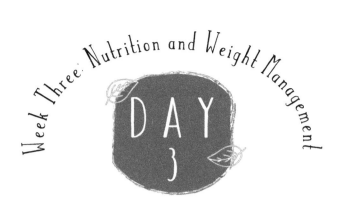

Week Three: Nutrition and Weight Management

DAY 3

KEY PRINCIPLES FOR WEIGHT MANAGEMENT

I enter today's discussion knowing the topic of weight management is a sore subject for some. Perhaps when you were in middle school, your mother often commented on your "round cheeks" or "sturdy" frame. Maybe you have been or are currently involved in a relationship with a man who jokes about your weight. Or maybe as you gathered measurements yesterday, you remembered a battle with anorexia or bulimia and fear returning to old ways should you give weight too much thought.

In the preface of this study, I shared that in childhood I tended to overeat. And boy, were my peers quick to comment on it! If I close my eyes and allow my mind to wander back, I know their words and the feelings associated with them can still haunt me. That's why I refuse to think on things that discourage (see Philippians 4:8). Instead, when it comes to the subjects of managing my weight and how I view myself as I work on the matter, I remember what God's Word says about me:

> [God] shaped me first inside, then out; [He] formed me in my
> mother's womb. I thank you, High God—you're breathtaking!
> Body and soul, I am marvelously made! I worship in
> adoration—what a creation! You know me inside and out,
> you know every bone in my body; You know exactly how I
> was made, bit by bit, how I was sculpted from nothing into
> something. Like an open book, you watched me grow from
> conception to birth; all the stages of my life were spread out
> before you, The days of my life all prepared before I'd even
> lived one day. (Psalm 139:13–16 MSG)

Don't forget that this passage is just as applicable to you as it was to the psalmist. We must not lose sight of the truth that we are designer's originals who are precious to the Lord.

God is so much more than our vinedresser. He is the master potter, and we humans are clay in His hands. He shapes us and molds us according to His plans (see Isaiah 64:8). Whether we are tall and thin or short and stout, we are individually designed with care and purpose. And as we talk more about weight management today, don't for a second allow yourself to think that ideal is unattainable for you because you have a certain body type or because you have an overactive metabolism. Friend, it would be boring if we all looked the same! God has shaped and formed each of us in creative, breathtaking ways. Remember that our goal in getting a handle on keys to weight management is not uniformity. We aim for wellness and a deeper respect for the unique temples God designed for us.

Key Principles for Managing Weight

Below are six simple principles for weight management that can be easily incorporated into the way we care for our temples. As you read, place a check mark beside those you are already doing. Put an exclamation point beside the one change you'd most like to adopt.

1   **Don't diet; make healthy eating a lifestyle.** Few of us like the thought of dieting, depriving ourselves of flavorful favorites in hopes of hitting a number on the scale. It's far more appealing to make small adjustments to the way we eat so weight management feels more natural and less threatening to our comfort. So (1) make it your goal to continue eating foods you enjoy. Just learn to prepare them in healthy ways or to limit yourself to one serving size instead of two. (2) Remember there is no need to starve. Have healthy 100-calorie snack packs and favorite fresh produce available at home and work—and even in the car for when you are on the go. And (3) if possible, eat five to six smaller meals each day rather than the standard big three. Eating every few hours will help you stay full and less prone to overdoing. All these adjustments can lead to big changes without the pain of traditional dieting.

2   **Remember that variety is a friend.** Few like to eat the same thing day after day. Each week we should branch out and try a new fruit or veggie. When we plan meals—a topic we'll discuss in more detail in day 5—we should try to incorporate a variety of colors into our selection of vegetables. We may also find it helpful to get creative with our snack choices. This week, for instance, I'm trying bell peppers of all colors on Monday, a spoonful of almond butter on Tuesday, a small package of almonds on Wednesday, and some yogurt and granola on Thursday. Ideally, we want to consume foods that not only are good for us but also will keep us full. That principle applies to snacks and meals.

3   **Know that fast food and many packaged snacks will work against you.** Drive-through meals are quick lunch options, and a big box of snack cakes or a bag of cheesy chips can easily soothe cravings—for a while. But foods like these are notoriously high in fat. And when it comes to consuming options like these, we usually give little thought to proper portion size. Accessing such foods, in fact, often turns into a temptation to overeat! By not eating fried foods, sugary snacks, or fatty fast food products, you can eliminate many

saturated and trans fats and a lot of excess calories. This will lead to a healthier you.

4. **Slow down and enjoy your meals.** How easy it is to sit down at a Mexican restaurant, gorge on chips and salsa, and then stuff ourselves on huge entrées! In our culture, if the food is in front of us, it seems we must eat all of it—and do so as quickly as we can.

A much wiser approach to mealtime involves preparation. It involves drinking a six- to eight- ounce glass of water to take the edge off our hunger before we eat. When we dine out, we should consider selecting an item or two from the *a la carte* menu to avoid feeling we must eat enough to justify the expense. And when we begin to eat, whether at home or elsewhere, we must pace ourselves. Chewing each bite sixteen to twenty times aids digestion and helps us avoid overeating. Should we finish our food and find we are still hungry, we might choose a small salad or side of fruit instead of dessert.

5. **Avoid empty calorie consumption.** We should never waste our daily calorie intake on sugary sodas and fruit drinks, popular though these products may be. Water and healthy teas are far better options. An added bonus is that staying hydrated keeps our skin more supple and can improve our complexion. It also helps us avoid nighttime dry mouth and leads to better sleep.

6. **Don't discount the value of exercise.** Humans were not meant to sit at desks all day. And the steady supply of high-calorie food Americans eat on top of our often-sedentary jobs sets us up for weight issues. The American Heart Association encourages us to exercise thirty minutes five times a week[9]—a goal that is just as well reached if we perform activities for ten to fifteen minutes, two or three times a day for five days. Either way, each of us should have a

---

9   "American Heart Association Recommendations for Physical Activity in Adults." Posted February 2014. *American Heart Association:* http://www.heart.org/HEARTORG/HealthyLiving/ PhysicalActivity/FitnessBasics/American-Heart-Association-Recommendations- for-Physical-Activity-in-Adults_UCM_307976_Article.jsp#.V5eog2VGi-I (July 26, 2016).

weekly plan to reach 150 minutes of get-out-of-the-chair-and-get-moving exercise.

Determining that movement—whether we are walking or working out at the gym— will be a fabulous tool for weight management.

Reflections

What did you find most helpful about today's lesson? Why?

_____

_____

_____

_____

Daily Exercise Prompt

Go for a fifteen-minute walk or bike ride today, and do a bit of stretching when you finish. As you work, think about ways you can implement the six principles of weight management.

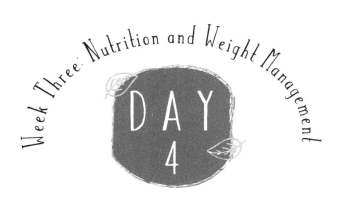

Week Three: Nutrition and Weight Management

DAY 4

AVOIDING OBSESSION, CHOOSING MODERATION

As you begin working to apply the weight management principles we discussed yesterday, I want to visit the necessity of self-control in making healthy changes. It's an important tool in preventing obsession.

The concept of self-control is not just a spiritual fruit (one that I like to envision as a delectable strawberry). It is also an idea based on "the Greek word *enkrateia*, which means . . . restraining passions and appetites."[10] Biblically speaking, the proper attitude of the believer is one of self-control over all desires. Interestingly, in classical Greek, self-control was a sign of human freedom: "One was truly free if he could control his desire for . . . food."[11]

Based on that statement, would you say you are truly free, somewhat free, or enslaved to physical appetites? Explain your answer.

_____

10   Gilbrant, *The Complete Biblical Library*, 212.

11   Ibid.

_____

_____

_____

_____

In her study *Living Beyond Yourself*, author Beth Moore offered this insight: "It is not God's will for us to be mastered by anything other than HIM. God wants us to be free from obsession: from the obsession of eating and from the obsession of not eating."[12] If we allow dreams of food or even calorie-counting to take over our thoughts, we risk falling into the trap Moore warns against. We risk making food (or maybe even keeping fit in general) an idol of sorts—something that competes for the focus and dedication that belong to God alone.

It may seem odd that I'm linking the good decision to make healthy choices with idolatry. Please don't misunderstand—taking care of ourselves is a good thing. But I want to be careful not to leave you with the impression that it should be our most important thing. Pursuing physical wellness deserves balanced focus, not wholehearted devotion.

Healthy eating is about intentional daily moderation; it's about avoiding extremes. Moderation looks like eating five to six times a day from a small plate of healthy selections.

If over the course of the next few weeks you find yourself growing anxious over mealtime or grocery shopping, it's time to take a break from this study and instead immerse yourself in the Word. And remember the wisdom of the apostle Paul: "Physical training [whether that includes counting calories or running laps] is of some value, but godliness has value for all things, holding

---

12   Beth Moore, *Living Beyond Yourself: Exploring the Fruit of the Spirit*. (Nashville: Life Way Press, 2007), 119.

promise for both the present life and the life to come" (1 Timothy 4:8). We should desire a growing relationship with the Lord above all else.

Precious sister in Christ, I am praying you will love to feast on God's Word and will choose to consume the nutritious foods He has created just for you in the way that is best. By all means, make the changes necessary to make your temple as physically fit as possible. But remember: it's your spiritual health that is of ultimate value.

Reflections

What if anything about today's lesson challenged you?

_____

_____

_____

_____

Daily Exercise Prompt

Go for a fifteen-minute walk, jog, or swim today, and do a bit of stretching when you finish. As you work, reflect on the Beth Moore quote: "It is not God's will for us to be mastered by anything other than HIM."[13]

---

13   Ibid.

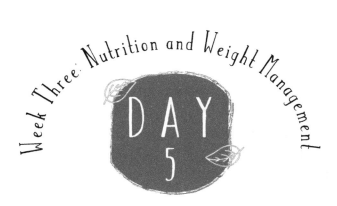

FILLING THE FRIDGE AND PANTRY

Over my years of teaching health and wellness, I've heard repeatedly that one of the most challenging parts of eating properly is *preparing* to eat properly. Today's content is designed as a plan of action. It's meant to provide tips and tools that can make grocery shopping a pleasant experience that supports healthy eating.

First, let's talk basics. You may remember seeing a food pyramid with six basic food groups in your high school textbook. The categories were listed in the order of serving sizes recommended for daily consumption. The smallest group—fats, oils, and sweets—sat atop the pyramid and was to be consumed sparingly. The group on the bottom consisted of bread, rice, cereal, and pasta; these were the foods meant to be consumed most often. The foods in the middle—fruits and veggies and proteins—were to be eaten regularly and in moderation. This food pyramid is an old model and now obsolete.

A newer personalized version of the revised concept may be found on wellness sites such as https://www.choosemyplate.gov and https://www. eatright.org. I discovered as a woman of my size with a medium body frame, I need to consume around 2,000 calories a day to maintain my recommended weight.[14] In terms of healthy consumption, the site informs me that this means I need about three cups of vegetables, six ounces of grains, two and a half cups of fruit, five cups of protein, three cups of dairy, and no more than five ounces of oils and sweets daily. I also need to consume about sixty-five ounces of water per day.

I share all this because consuming the kind of well-rounded meals our bodies need requires that we think carefully about what we'll eat rather than moving throughout our days with no plan and grabbing whatever sounds good in the moment. Below is a list of helpful principles to keep in mind before we start preparing for a run to the grocery store.

1. Breakfast is the most important meal of the day, so don't skip it. A hearty first meal gets the metabolism going.

2. Eating in saves money and leads to better portion control.

3. Water is usually the best choice of drink, and it's a big money-saver. Flavoring it can help make drinking water more appealing.

4. The last meal of the day should be the lightest meal of the day. And the later you sit down to eat, the lighter that meal should be. (Six o'clock is a good goal.)

5. Though there's no need to eat dessert daily, learning to substitute a light option like Jell-O® and Cool Whip Lite® for a big slice of chocolate cake can satisfy a sweet tooth.

6. Portion size is no joke. If you tend to overload your plate, it's time to buy dinnerware that has a decreased circumference.

---

14   Personalize your own meal plans and cuisine experiences by using one or both of these websites: https://www.choosemyplate.gov and https://www.eatright.org

/ Going to the grocery store without a list is just as dangerous as going there hungry. Always, always prepare for the excursion.

Using the information I've included above as well as peeking at the recommendations found at one of the above websites I created a meal plan for this week. You'll see that the plan carefully catalogs everything I want to make for the next seven days.

	Breakfast	Lunch	Dinner
MONDAY MEALS	Steel-cut oatmeal, fruit in season, low-fat milk	Salad with grilled chicken, decaf green tea	Baked salmon, kale and spring mix salad, water with lime
TUESDAY MEALS	Grain cereal, fruit, low-fat milk	Turkey sandwich on whole-grain bread with red-tip lettuce, tomato, water with lemon juice	Grilled chicken edamame, mixed spring salad with tomatoes, decaf green tea
WEDNESDAY MEALS	Grain English muffin, 2 egg whites scrambled with spinach, decaf coffee or skim milk	Low-sodium chicken breast on wrap with tomato and 2 tsp. hummus, water with lime juice	Crock-Pot® beef with lots of fresh veggies included, decaf white tea
THURSDAY MEALS	Two hard-boiled eggs with fresh fruit, unsweetened vanilla almond milk	Turkey burger on green-tip lettuce with veggies, 2 tsp. hummus, 1 tbsp. avocado, decaf flavored tea	Chicken kabobs, onions, bell pepper, squash, zucchini fresh green beans, water flavored with fruit
FRIDAY MEALS	Breakfast wrap with scrambled egg whites in whole-grain tortilla, salsa, bell peppers, skim milk or decaf coffee	Fish tacos with salsa and veggies, decaf green tea	Grilled halibut, grilled asparagus, decaf flavored tea
SATURDAY MEALS	Blueberry protein smoothie	Grilled chicken over spring mix, water with fruit	Stir fry veggies in peanut oil with brown rice, water with lime
SUNDAY MEALS	One cup steel-cut oatmeal with blueberries	Mediterranean salad with crunchy chickpeas, water with lemon	Tomato stuffed with chicken salad, fresh fruit, decaf green tea

Diagram E

Once I have this plan, I'm prepared to make my grocery list. One meal at a time, I write down every ingredient I'll need to make each meal. After that, at the bottom of the page I write down a few ideas for healthy snack options that can keep me full between times. So before we get into the meal plan, let's think about what kind of treats we will allow ourselves this week.

Circle the snack ideas that appeal to you. Remember: snacks should be around 100 calories.

celery and carrot sticks   yogurt with granola   small cherry tomatoes

a serving of almonds, walnuts, pecans   cucumber with hummus   a half cup of mixed berries

hard-boiled egg   one cup of steamed edamame in the shell   four tablespoons crunchy chickpeas

Now use the chart on the following page to create your own meal plan. Just for fun, I've included with each day a chore chart meant to get the family involved in dividing and conquering mealtime chores. Feel free to fill it in too.

Use your meal plan—and the snack ideas you circled above—to make a grocery list either on your smart phone or on a piece of paper.

	Breakfast	Lunch	Dinner
MONDAY MEALS			
Preparing the meal			
Setting the table			
Serving the food			
Cleaning up			
TUESDAY MEALS			
Preparing the food			
Setting the table			
Serving the food			
Cleaning up			
WEDNESDAY MEALS			
Preparing the food			
Setting the table			
Serving the food			
Cleaning up			
THURSDAY MEALS			
Preparing the food			
Setting the table			
Serving the food			
Cleaning up			
FRIDAY MEALS			
Preparing the food			
Setting the table			
Serving the food			
Cleaning up			

Diagram F

SATURDAY MEALS			
Preparing the meal			
Setting the table			
Serving the food			
Cleaning up			
SUNDAY MEALS			
Preparing the meal			
Setting the table			
Serving the food			
Cleaning up			

Before you head to the grocery store, decide which items would be best purchased at your local farmer's market. Organic, home-grown fruits and veggies, pasture-raised chicken and eggs, and even local cheeses often taste so much better than what we find in stores. If you want to make a stop at the farmer's market this week, divide your list into two.

Now you're almost ready to shop. Grab your coupons and keys, and keep in mind these shopping tips from dietician Sheila Kelly of *healthination.com*:

1   **It's best to shop the outer perimeter of your standard grocery store.** That's where you will find the healthiest food items: produce, proteins, and dairy. Packaged foods within the inner aisles often contain lots of preservatives and are high in sodium, low in fiber, and loaded with calories and sugar.

2   **Remember to make selections with colors and seasons in mind.** Try to purchase fresh vegetables in a variety of bright, deep colors. Familiarize yourself with what's in season, and feel free to ask your grocer for insight. It is cheaper to buy vegetables, fruits, and nuts when they are in season. Many vegetables are grown year round.

} **Know that frozen fruits and veggies are okay.** Just try to avoid things that have lots of added preservatives: check your labels. It's particularly important to watch out for fruit that may have been packed with lots of sugar. If selecting a frozen yogurt treat, look for items that are low in fat or fat-free.

4. **Don't steer clear of the dairy aisle.** Today's dairy case has many low-fat and/or fat-free items, including lactose-free products. Butter substitutes like liquid or tub margarine are better choices than stick butter or margarine that contains a lot of bad fats.

5 **Take care in your selection of meats.** Deli meat is notoriously loaded with sodium. Use discretion at the deli counter. Select only lean meats with low sodium and no preservatives. If purchasing ground beef, select a package labeled 96 percent fat free. If buying fish, avoid breading or stuffing. If chicken or turkey is on your list, select white, skinless meat.[15]

There's one more bit of information I want you to have as you wander those aisles. Food labels can take some of the confusion out of shopping. When you grab a package or can, flip it over to see the serving size of that product. Note that whatever calorie count is given for that product usually applies to only one serving.

To find healthy foods, it is important to take a good, long look at each label. It will give you an idea of what and how much is hiding in the product. Check your serving sizes. Does this item contain one, two, or more servings? Do you recognize the ingredients listed on the label? Most manufacturers will list ingredients in declining order. The first item you read under that heading is always the main ingredient in the product. It's a good rule of thumb to look at the first three items listed. If you are not familiar with them or they contain words like *hydrogenated* or *shortening* or words ending with *-ose* (sucrose,

---

15   Sheila Kelly, *"Healthy Grocery Shopping: Fresh Foods."* Posted March 2, 2016. *HealthiNation:* Sheila Kelly, *"Healthy Grocery Shopping"* retrieved February 7, 2017. HealthiNation: https://www.healthination. com/nutrition-essentials/test-31-preview/healthy-grocery-shopping-fresh-foods-1/ (July 26, 2016).

dextrose, and so on), chances are you would be better off not buying that product.

You can also go to Healthination.com to the nutrition area to find more ideas on how to choose and purchase healthy food items and to read labels.

Reflections

What if anything about today's lesson challenged you to shop for healthier food items? Explain.

_____

_____

_____

_____

_____

Daily Exercise Prompt

Take your list of healthy foods, and park as far as you can from the front door of your market. Walk briskly into the store. Once inside, continue to walk the perimeter as well as up and down each aisle before grabbing a cart. Then as you shop, don't hesitate to reach high and stoop low to reach for your purchases.

Week Four

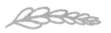

MOVING FOR CHANGE

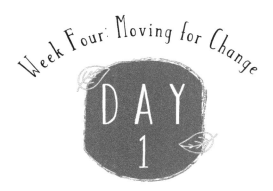

Week Four: Moving for Change

DAY 1

THE HEART'S SPIRITUAL IMPORTANCE

Much of this week's content will revolve around caring for the literal hearts that beat within our chests. However, "in the King James Version of the Bible the word 'heart' is mentioned in the Old Testament 725 times and 105 times in the New Testament. That is a total of 830 times [the] heart is referred to in the Bible."[1] Most of those references speak of the heart in its spiritual sense, so let's begin our discussion of this vital organ by considering it in that capacity.

Biblically speaking, the heart is the core and center of who we really are. "As a face is reflected in water," Proverbs 27:19 states, "so the heart reflects the real person" (NLT). The heart is the part of us that God, our vinedresser, "searches" (Romans 8:27). It is the part He evaluates, for it is our heart that reveals our true character (1 Samuel 16:7). Moreover, the stuff we cherish within our hearts most influences the words and attitudes that come from our mouth. "Whatever is in your heart," Matthew 12:34 notes, "determines what you say" (NLT).

---

1   Cliff Leitch, ed., "Word Counts: How Many Times Does a Word Appear in the Bible?" *Christian Bible Reference Site: http://www.christianbiblereference.org/faq_WordCount.htm* (August 3, 2016).

The Greek definition of the word *kardia*, for *heart*, gives additional insight. *Heart* obtains its origins "as the seat of the desires, feelings, affections, passions . . . to say 'in one's heart' means to think . . . to place or keep in the heart means to lay up or keep in one's mind. . . . In the New Testament the heart represents especially the sphere of God's influence in the human life."[2]

Perhaps no biblical biography better highlights the importance of the heart in a spiritual sense than that of David—shepherd, giant slayer, and eventual king over Israel. We first meet young David when the prophet Samuel shows up at his Bethlehem home to anoint one of Jesse's sons as king. No sooner does Samuel arrive than he is impressed by the size and the handsome face of Jesse's oldest boy, Eliab. *Surely this guy is the Lord's anointed!* Samuel thought at the sight of him. But God stopped Samuel with these words: "Do not consider his appearance or his height, for I have rejected him. The Lord does not look at the things people look at. People look at the outward appearance, but the Lord looks at the heart" (1 Samuel 16:7). God, we learn, is not nearly as concerned with the way a person looks on the outside as He is with the way a person looks on the inside.

> ***What about you? Do you typically draw conclusions about people based on what you see on their outside—or based on what you know about the condition of their heart? Provide an example to illustrate.***

_____

_____

_____

_____

When David's story continues in 1 Samuel 17, it's not long before we get some clues about what was going on in Eliab's heart and what kinds of things led God to reject him as king over the Israelites. After David is anointed Israel's

---

2   Spiros Zodhiates and Warren Patrick Baker, eds., *Hebrew-Greek Key Word Study Bible NIV*. New Testament Lexical Aids. (Chattanooga, TN: AMG Publishers, 1996), 1637.

next monarch and returns to shepherding until God's plan for him would further unfold, Eliab—who witnessed Samuel blessing David as his nation's next ruler—has felt only contempt for his youngest brother. As Eliab and the older brothers, serving as soldiers in King Saul's army, hear the threats of the Philistine warrior Goliath boom across the valley, David arrives to deliver food supplies from home. Listening to Goliath's words, the young David grows eager to go out and fight the man "who dares to defy the armies of Israel" because David knows "the God who delivered him from the paw of the lion and the paw of the bear" could also deliver the giant into his hands. Meanwhile, the physically impressive and handsome Eliab cowers under the giant's taunt. But he stands tall when it comes to insulting God's anointed: he puts David down, calls him names, and accuses David of just standing around to watch when he should be hurrying back to the sheep (1 Samuel 17:28).

David, however, is clearly a man devoted to God. The book of Psalms is filled with songs of praise he wrote to honor Him. And while I could bring out many other points relevant to this discussion, I'll focus on David's words after he had committed a terrible sin in his middle-age years: "Create in me a pure heart, O God, and renew a steadfast spirit in me" (Psalm 51:10). (Isn't that beautiful?) David, it seems, knew the value of allowing the Lord to rule his spiritual heart, to shape the very core of who he was in such a way that the Creator was glorified and others were blessed. Perhaps this is why God described David like this: he is "a man after my own heart; he will do everything I want him to do" (Acts 13:22).

Think of your heart in terms of this story. Would you say your spiritual heart is more like that of Eliab or David? Explain your answer.

_____

_____

_____

_____

Maybe you are living so wholeheartedly for the Lord that you didn't hesitate to equate your heart with David's. If so, that's wonderful! But if you are like me, you realized as you answered that question that you have some Eliab-like tendencies. If you do, be encouraged. Our God is in the heart-changing business.

What kinds of things should be spilling out of a Christ follower's heart?

_____

_____

_____

I hope you listed the fruit of the Spirit earlier. (Can you tell that I hope you'll memorize these?) As we know, God's power at work within us can transform even the crankiest Eliab into a devoted, kind servant like David.

The character trait we have chosen for heart issues this week is the Greek word *chrestotes* (both e's long) for *kindness*. *Chrestotes* is "useful, profitable, kindness, usefulness . . . the grace which prevails the whole nature, mellowing all which would be harsh and austere. . . . The word is descriptive of one's disposition . . ."[3] You have seen David demonstrating all these traits. Earlier on the horn of plenty diagram (p. 37), I selected the tomato and avocado to represent the spiritual fruit of kindness—which should be a hallmark character trait linked with all believers in Jesus. A red tomato cut in two has four separate chambers like what we see within a human heart. Avocadoes, full of fats and oils that are good for the physical heart, have an outer shell and soft flesh that hide a pit that can be planted to produce new avocado trees. Avocadoes, then, remind us that what is hidden within the hearts of in-love-with-Jesus Christians has great potential for good. It can lead to a harvest of righteousness.

---

3   Ibid., 1687.

Which of the following are kindnesses with which you could bless others, provided you allow the Holy Spirit to produce this trait in your heart? Star your selections.

Giving to the missions offering so people around the world can hear the gospel

Telling everyone who'll listen what you don't like about the pastor's sermon

Speaking encouragingly to others

Hoarding wealth

Providing food to the hungry

Offering to cover a shift for a coworker so she can spend time with her sick son

Taking time to prepare healthful meals for you and your family

Doing kind things began with God. What kindness He showed in offering us the plan of salvation though we don't deserve it! What kindness He shows us as He provides us with many great foods to eat, with families and friends, and with all the beauties of nature. Out of God's deep affection and love for His creation, He has kindly allowed you and me to be part of His kingdom!

When we get these truths deep down in our spiritual hearts, we cannot help but want to tell the Lord, "Thank You" by growing in Him and by taking every possible opportunity to extend kindness to others.

Reflections

What about today's discussion most resonated with you? Why?

_____

_____

_____

_____

Daily Exercise Prompt

It's time to get that physical heart pumping! Today go on a twenty-minute walk or jog. As you move, think about ways God has been kind to you, and consider how you can share kindness with others. Make it your goal to do one particularly kind thing for a neighbor, coworker, or family member before your next lesson. Don't forget to stretch when you complete your workout.

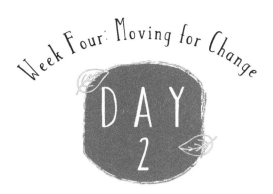

Week Four: Moving for Change

DAY 2

THE PHYSICAL HEART AND
HOW TO TRAIN IT

Our physical heart, the centerpiece of our circulatory system, is one of the largest muscles within our temple. It rhythmically contracts, serving as a blood pump that circulates life-giving nutrients throughout our body. The heart is responsible for distributing oxygen, carbon dioxide, nutrients, and hormones necessary for maintaining proper cell function throughout our temple. Evaluating heart health, then, can provide many insights into one's health in general.

During an annual physical, your doctor will likely take a sample of your blood, check your blood pressure, and may even administer a stress test or EKG. The results of these tests can help your physician determine whether you have a strong, healthy heart or one suffering with a blockage or a disease.

In week 2, day 3, alongside the Strong Temple Stylish Information we collected, I discussed what kinds of things are revealed when we submit to laboratory blood work. I also introduced the blood pressure concept, but let's talk about that in more depth here. Remember: a blood pressure measurement involves two numbers, and 120 over 80 is the norm. The first, or top, number is called the systolic blood pressure. It measures the pressure at which your blood is being pushed against the walls of your arteries during the forceful contraction (or systole phase) of a typical heartbeat. The lower, or bottom, number is a measure of the intensity of your blood's travel back to the heart during that organ's relaxation phase. This is called diastole or diastolic blood pressure.

To put this information into practical use, recall your most recent blood pressure results, and measure your heart's wellness against the following recommendations provided by the American Heart Association.[4]

Blood Pressure Chart

This blood pressure chart reflects categories defined by the American Heart Association.

Blood Pressure Category	Systolic mm Hg (upper #)		Diastolic mm Hg (lower #)
Normal	less than 120	and	less than 80
Prehypertension	120 – 139	or	80 – 89
High Blood Pressure (Hypertension) Stage 1	140 – 159	or	90 – 99
High Blood Pressure (Hypertension) Stage 2	160 or higher	or	100 or higher
Hypertensive Crisis (Emergency care needed)	Higher than 180	or	Higher than 110

Your doctor should evaluate unusually low or high readings.

Diagram G

---

4   "Understanding Blood Pressure Readings." *American Heart Association:* http://www.heart.org/HEARTORG/Conditions/HighBloodPressure/AboutHighBloodPressure/ Understanding-Blood-Pressure- Readings_UCM_301764_Article.jsp?gclid=CNW2x-WCyMoCFQGTaQodHhUCjw#.VqevdfkrLlU (August 3, 2016).

What do you notice about the overall health of your heart?

_____

_____

_____

I hope you were able to note, based on the information in the chart, that you have a healthy heart, which can lead to your enjoyment of many years as you continue to pursue a high-quality, active lifestyle. It could be, however, that you detect—as your doctor would if he or she were to do the same test—evidence of disease in your heart. High blood pressure can be a strong indicator that high cholesterol and fat have led to blocked arteries. This often presents itself as prehypertension or hypertension, and left unaddressed, it can contribute to cardiovascular disease (CVD)—commonly called by names like "stroke" and "heart attack."

The great news is that even if you find yourself in the danger zone for encountering such issues, you are already on the path to making corrective measures. A healthier diet, as we have discussed extensively already, leads to a healthier heart. And cardio or aerobic activity, in which I just know you have been engaging since at least the start of our time together, is excellent preventative maintenance for this valuable organ. Cardio exercise rushes oxygen to the heart, strengthens it over time, and eventually decreases how hard the heart must work whether you are running a marathon or are sitting and reading a book.

In scanning the title of this week's content, you may have groaned at the thought of my asking more of you physically than I have so far. The idea of "moving for change" may not get you as excited as it does me. My prayer is that by the time you finish this week of content, you will decide once and for all that rather than being discouraged by exercise, you will see it as an opportunity to invest in you and in the future of those you love. Temple maintenance really can be fun!

Time to TRAIN

For this next section of our study, I am incorporating the teachings of my friend Dr. J., with whom I co-wrote the men's version of this book. Below we present TRAIN for basic cardio. Simply put, TRAIN consists of five basic principles that can take the confusion and the overwhelming sensation out of exercising so we can enjoy it.

TRAIN stands for **t**ype of exercise, **r**acing the clock, **a**ccountability, **i**ntensity of the exercise, and the **n**umber of days a particular activity is done.

> "The type of exercise" refers simply to the specific activities you can do to get moving. Cardio exercises such as walking, jogging, and swimming, aerobics, and so on are better for getting the heart in shape. Others, such as weight training and calisthenics, are better for making the muscles strong. Consider that even participation in sports—whether that means playing tennis, racquetball, or softball, or even making the rounds at a golf course—are all good ways to get fit.
>
> The phrase "racing the clock" is a reminder that the amount of time spent in exercise will determine the benefits received. In general, the longer you exercise, the more benefit your heart gets. This is true up to a point; one can overdo it. Exercising at least thirty minutes a day five days a week is a great goal.
>
> "Accountability" is critical to persevering in a plan to develop and maintain wellness. The individuals who come alongside you while you seek to improve your health have the potential to assure your success or failure.

"Intensity," represented by the "I" in TRAIN, refers to how hard an exercise should be done to achieve the best results. Exercise should not be too intense, or the body will suffer consequences that work against it. Similarly, not exercising with enough intensity will lead to frustration over the lack of improvement. So what is the right intensity? The Talk Test can help us find it.

Simply stated, if you can talk during exercise, you are generally at the right intensity. If you can sing or whistle while you go about it, you are not working hard enough. If you are having trouble breathing while trying to communicate, you are likely working too hard.

The Talk Test

1   Stand up and stretch lightly before you begin slowly jogging or exercise in place to warm up.

2   Try to sing or whistle a few bars of your favorite song as you move. If you find that easy to do, you are moving too slowly to receive much heart benefit from the exercise.

3   Increase your pace. As you do, recite a Scripture verse or the lyrics to a favorite song. If you can speak and move without feeling overly winded, you've found a good pace.

4   Increase your speed until you feel your heart thumping. Try to recite something simple, such as the Lord's Prayer, as you do. If you find it difficult to speak and exercise at the same time, it's likely you need to slow down to avoid injury.

5   Slow your pace down to a walk, lightly stretch, and sit down.

Finally, the "number of days" referenced by TRAIN refers to the frequency with which an exercise is repeated. Some exercises, such as the walking we do every day just to get around, may be done without much thought as to their recurrence. Other exercises, such as aerobics, jogging, swimming, and so on will require some rest and recuperation between times for best effects to be achieved. Although some experts hold that exercise should be done daily, our stance is that each of us needs at least one weekly day of rest from all exercise to allow our temples to perform at their best."[5]

More Self-Monitoring

I'd like to cover one more topic before I close. Pulse-monitoring, like the Talk Test Dr. J. mentioned, is another excellent tool for measuring how hard you are—or are not—exercising.

You can check your own pulse easily at the carotid artery, which runs down your neck an inch or so away from the center of your throat. To get an accurate measurement of the palpable beat of your heart as blood expands your circulatory system, sit comfortably for about 15 to 20 minutes before checking your resting heart rate. Then place your index and middle finger on the side of your neck and feel for your heartbeat. Once you locate it, count the number of times you feel your pulse in a 15-second period; you will need a timer to do this effectively. Multiply that number by four to get your estimated pulse. (For adults, the normal resting heart rate is sixty to one hundred beats per minute.)

---

5   Wayne Jacobs with Kathryn Baker, *The Strong Temple: A Man's Guide to Developing Spiritual and Physical Health.* (Bloomington, IN: Westbow Press, 2015), 22–27.

Let's try it now while you are close to a resting heart rate.
How many beats did you count within fifteen seconds? _____

Multiply that number by four to find your pulse rate.
Write it here: _____

> "Generally," my colleague points out, "a lower resting heart rate indicates more efficient heart function and better cardiovascular fitness. For example, an athlete might have a normal resting heart rate between 40 to 50 beats a minute. In other words, the lower a pulse rate is, the less the heart has to work. That is because when a heart is stronger, it can pump more blood with each beat."[6]

Now, get up and run in place for approximately two minutes.
Check your pulse again, writing your heart rate here: _____

What happened to your pulse rate after this activity?

_____

You probably saw that your heart rate increased when you got up and began moving. "Consider," Dr. Jacobs says, "that when a heart rate is high when resting, the organ must pound even more intensely to compensate for any exertion. The feeling that accompanies this phenomenon, however, is not something to be used as an excuse not to exercise. In time, regular exertion leads to a lower resting pulse rate, which is far better for the heart and body and also proves more comfortable during exercise."[7] To illustrate his point, I've provided the following example:

---

6   Ibid., 21.
7   Ibid., 22.

Gloria has a resting heart rate of sixty beats per minute (bpm); Elie Jo's resting heart rate is seventy-five bpm. This means Gloria's heart beats significantly fewer times than Elie Jo's. If we compare the total number of beats for both women, we see something striking:

	Beats per Hour	Beats per Day	Beats per Year
Gloria	3,600	86,400	31,536,000
Elie Jo	4,500	108,000	39,420,000
Difference	900	21,600	7,884,000

Elie Jo's heart beats almost eight million more times in a year than Gloria's! If we extend that out over seventy years, Elie Jo's heart will have beaten at least 551,880,000 more times than Gloria's. Do you see the story of wear and tear at work here? Indeed, all those extra "resting" beats contribute to the mechanics of a circulatory system wearing out early.

Reflections

What about today's discussion do you most wish to remember?

_____

_____

Daily Exercise Prompt

Tomorrow we will establish a TRAIN cardio exercise plan together. In the meantime, spend at least twenty minutes today on cardio activities we've tried so far that can help get that heart (or keep it) in top shape. Don't forget to incorporate stretches from Appendix B. (Bonus points if you try something new!)

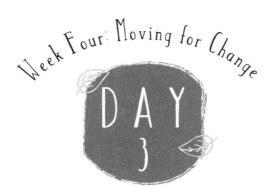

Week Four: Moving for Change

DAY 3

ESTABLISHING A CARDIO EXERCISE ROUTINE

I am so excited that by the end of today's lesson you will have a basic personalized training plan you can begin putting into effect immediately. If you read that line with anything less than enthusiasm, let me share this verse of encouragement that can help you move forward with a positive outlook.

> **Read the following Bible passage aloud: "Whatever you do, work at it with all your heart, as working for the Lord" (Colossians 3:23).**

Remember: getting in shape is part of caring for the temples God has given us. When we are in good health, we have more energy for doing the good works He has prepared for us. So please determine with me that you will jump into today's lesson with a positive attitude and a determination to be your best you for God's glory. It's time to be kind to your heart!

Fill in the exercise prescription below, remembering that the pursuit of wellness will require you to work out for a total of 150 minutes weekly. At this point, please select only one activity.

My Basic Cardio TRAINing Prescription

I plan to implement this *type* of cardio exercise: _____

_____, by *racing the clock* for _____ minutes at a time. I will ask _____ to partner with me for the sake of *accountability*. I will faithfully use the Talk Test to monitor the *intensity* of my workout, making adjustments as needed. The *number of days* I will work out each week is _____.[8]

Responses to this will vary, but maybe you said you would start running five days a week for thirty minutes at a time, looking to your husband to hold you accountable. That is a great goal, but remember that you may need to work up to it—especially if you are going from a sedentary lifestyle to one that includes such a rigorous routine. Taking baby steps in the right direction will still get you to your destination.

Now let's take the information from your prescription and convert it into a chart to tack onto the wall where you will see it regularly.

For you to see how easily this chart can be adapted as you develop a more complex weekly cardio routine, add at least one more exercise to it. It's okay to shorten one activity to accommodate a new one. (And remember—household chores like vacuuming or cleaning bathrooms count as exercise.)

---

8   Ibid., 27.

CARDIO TRAIN CHART

	Day1	Day 2	Day 3	Day 4	Day 5
T					
R					
A					
I					
N					

Chart H

The Need for Perseverance

I hope your TRAIN chart makes you eager to get up and active. But since everyone knows that many of the people who start off with great fitness resolutions at New Year's rarely keep them through March, I offer a word of caution. The plain truth is that most people lack the perseverance needed to continue in an exercise routine as life gets hectic and the newness wears off. While I could cite many articles offering helpful advice on avoiding this tendency as we make our own fitness plans, I will turn instead to one of my favorite verses in the Bible. I find it more motivating for staying the course than all the combined advice of health magazines.

Read Hebrews 12:1–3:

> Since we are surrounded by such a great cloud of witnesses, let us throw off everything that hinders and the sin that so easily entangles. And let us run with perseverance the race marked out for us, fixing our eyes on Jesus, the pioneer and perfecter of our faith. For the joy set before him he endured the cross, scorning its shame, and sat down at the right hand of the throne of God. Consider him who endured such opposition from sinners, so that you will not grow weary and lose heart.

In the original context of this verse, the apostle Paul likened the Christian's spiritual journey to a race. He talked about the importance of staying focused on Jesus, seeing Him as life's ultimate prize. Paul also spoke of life as if it is a thing that plays out before the eyes of many watching spectators. Bible scholars are divided over whether this passage refers to angelic witnesses or the heroes of faith who are now home with Christ. In either case, the idea is that we as Christians have a heavenly cheering section fixed on our spiritual progress and cheering us on. In a world rocked by the effects of sin, a determined eye on the prize of eternity with the Lord and a mind cheered by the facts can help us avoid losing heart and growing so discouraged that we give up.

When I read this passage, I see it first through the lens of this literal interpretation—as we should. But I also see within it some principles that help me to stay my fitness course. These verses remind me that people—whether my family or other ladies who face health struggles like mine—are watching me. The choices I make, then, are never made in a vacuum: they will impact others. With that in mind, I tap into new fuel for saying no to things like gluttony and laziness, which can take me off course. Those things are, after all, only sins that will entangle me. Further, I remember that in everything I do, pleasing Jesus is my ultimate goal. Keeping my temple fit is one way I try to honor Him.

The passage also reminds me that things worth doing are rarely easy. But just as sure as Christ did not grow so discouraged by the thought of the Passion ahead that He sidestepped the cross, I too must take care not to lose heart. If my Lord and Savior could do the hard things required of Him, surely with His help I can do the difficult things I set out to do. By establishing a routine and choosing perseverance, I'm well on my way to doing just that.

Reflections

What key words or concepts from today's material most spoke to you? Explain.

_____

_____

_____

_____

_____

_____

Daily Exercise Prompt

Today's the day to start putting that TRAIN chart to good use. With a goal of getting at least twenty minutes of exercising and some stretching in today, do the cardio activity of your choice. Try to get your routine in at least four hours before bedtime so the endorphins awakened during exercise have time to calm.

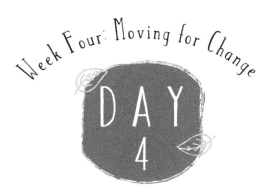

DAY 4

IDENTIFYING FUN AND CREATIVE WAYS TO GET ACTIVE

A young student once told me that horses sweat, men perspire, but ladies glow when exercising. I like the new perspective this brings to the idea of getting fit because as sure as perspiring doesn't have to *sound* like a bad thing, glowing from working out really can be fun! Today's lesson is all about finding new and unusual ways to get moving.

Think about your usual approach to life. How much priority do you typically place on remaining active?

High Priority   Some Priority   No Priority

Before we talk specifics, it's important to realize just how dangerous it is to allow our free time to become nothing more than an excuse to sit in front of the television set or gaming console, to text, to surf Facebook, or to play with an iPhone for hours on end. If most of your entertainment involves going to the movies or eating out, it's time to find some new hobbies—particularly if you have a desk job.

Whether we are checking email, creating, writing, or surfing online, those uninterrupted hours spent on our backsides can add up to serious health concerns. "Five or more hours of sedentary sitting," according to Dr. David Agus, who was interviewed by the *Chicago Tribune*, "is the health equivalent of smoking a pack and a quarter of cigarettes."[9]

The good news is that by making a few simple changes, we can lower some of the risks. Gretchen Reynolds, a reporter on exercise research for *The New York Times*, wrote a book condensing health studies to their most essential parts. One of the key takeaways from her research was this emphasis on standing up and the golden twenty-minute mark:

> New science shows very persuasively that standing up about every 20 minutes, even for only a minute or two, reduces your risk of developing diabetes and heart disease. By standing up, you cause the big muscles in your legs and back to contract, which leads to an increase in certain enzymes that break up fat in the blood stream. You don't have to jog in place or do jumping jacks. Just stand. A very pleasant additional benefit is that standing up every 20 to 30 minutes also seems to prompt the body to burn calories, so you don't gain as much weight from sitting at the office most of the day.[10]

---

9   Kevan Lee, "The Healthiest Way to Work: Standing vs. Sitting and Everything in Between." Posted September 4, 2014. *Chicago Tribune*: *http://www.chicagotribune.com/bluesky/hub/chi-buffer-healthiest-way-to-work-standing-vs-sitting-bsi-hub-story.html* (August 3, 2016).

10   Ibid.

Other studies confirm the benefit of this simple act of standing. For instance, a study of employees at New Balance shoe headquarters showed that performing an activity every thirty minutes—standing, walking, stretching—improved not only health but also engagement and concentration.[11]

So make sure you get up and move throughout your workday. As the American Health Association suggests, brainstorm project ideas with a coworker while taking a walk, stroll down the hall to speak with someone face-to-face rather than relying on messaging, take the stairs instead of the elevator, and request a stand-up desk.[12] Your heart and body will thank you.

The same basic principle should apply to the way we use our off hours. While there is certainly a time to rest or even to just relax in a hammock, we should work to stay in motion throughout the day and early evening.

Which of the following activities could you easily incorporate into your home time? Circle them.

working in the garden

mowing the grass

raking leaves

pruning trees

picking up trash

doing stretches during TV time

pedaling a stationary bicycle while listening to music

taking the dog for long walks

getting down on the floor and playing with the kids

throwing a football in the yard with your spouse or children

standing during phone calls

organizing drawers

running up and down the steps

---

11   Ibid.

12   "Get Moving! Easy Tips to Get Active." Posted September 2014. *American Heart Association*: http://www.heart.org/HEARTORG/HealthyLiving/PhysicalActivity/GettingActive/Get-Moving-Easy-Tips-to-Get- Active_UCM_307978_Article.jsp#.V5EvRGVGi-I (August 3, 2016).

Which activities could you pursue over the weekend? (Remember: a good change of scenery can stimulate the mind.)

hiking	window shopping	canoeing
cycling	sightseeing	paddle boarding
swimming	dancing	playing sports

All the above ideas are great ways to incorporate movement into your routine without having to label it exercise. These activities burn calories. They improve overall health. And many of them are just plain fun.

Reflections

Which of the above ideas for getting up and moving do you find most appealing?

_____

_____

_____

Daily Exercise Prompt

In addition to following your TRAIN chart and the related stretches you use for a cool-down, select an activity suggestion from today's lesson to incorporate into the remainder of your day.

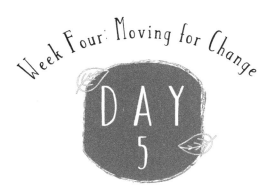

Week Four: Moving for Change

DAY 5

REMAINING ALERT TO SIGNS OF HEART DISEASE

Spiritual Heart Difficulties

When most people think of heart problems, they think in terms of diseases affecting the physical organ. But spiritual heart problems are just as deadly—perhaps even more so. That's why we'll begin today with a focus on them.

What behaviors do you think may indicate spiritual heart problems?

_____

_____

_____

Spiritual heart issues often show up in the form of sins like bitterness, deceit, foolishness, pride, arrogance, selfishness, lies, cheating, vengefulness, jealousy, and covetousness. (Eliab's story comes to mind.) The people of Judah offer another great scriptural example that gives insight into how these sins indicate a crippled heart. When they walked in obedience to God, they thrived in their land. When they attempted to do life without following God's law, they landed themselves in trouble. Over time, their hearts grew so jaded and hardened against right that they began thinking that whatever god they chose to serve would care for them. Sins like those listed above began to characterize Judah's people.

Eventually this collective and progressive heart condition left the people so blind to their faults and deaf to God's love for them that they saw no need to repent. Sinful behavior and wrong attitudes seemed the acceptable norm. But as their behavior grew worse and worse and hearts hardened more and more, a day came when the Lord handed them over to their Babylonian enemies. The people of Judah were carried off into exile. Many would never see their homeland again.

The Hebrew-Greek Key Word Study Bible correctly notes, "The most important thing in anybody's life is . . . having a heart that is 'right with God' (Acts 8:21)."[13] With this in mind, we better understand the promise God made to Ezekiel regarding His wayward, exiled people. He promised the Jews that a day would come when He would allow them to live in Judah again, and He would give them the help they needed to get back on track. "I'll give you a new heart. I'll put a new spirit in you. I'll cut out your stone heart and replace it with a red-blooded, firm-muscled heart. Then you'll obey my statutes and be careful to obey my commands. You'll be my people! I'll be your God!" (Ezekiel 11:18-19 MSG).

In Exodus 34:14 God is called a "jealous God" because He knows that only disappointment, hurt, and death await those who try to do life without Him. And He is a loving God who understands just how easy it is to allow our sinfully inclined hearts to wander into all kinds of problems. He wants us to obey, worship, and glorify Him—not just because He is worthy of our praise but also so we may have His blessing and enjoy the best lives possible. The

---

13   Zodhiates and Baker, *Hebrew-Greek Key Word Study Bible NIV*, 1637.

great news of Ezekiel 11 is that God has the power to soften our hearts and help us get back on track.

The condition of your spiritual heart is of great value to the Lord. So if you find yourself struggling with any heart issues, remember the truth of 1 John 1:9: "If we confess our sins, he is faithful and just and will forgive us our sins and purify us from all unrighteousness." He can "give [us] singleness of heart and action, so that [we] will always fear [Him] and that all will then go well for [us]" (Jeremiah 32:39).

Pause and write a prayer below, asking God to grant you a spiritually healthy heart. Be sure to include confession of sin.

_____

_____

_____

_____

Physical Heart Disease

Now that we have a better understanding of the spiritual disease that can invade our heart, let's talk about the two main forms of disease associated with our physical hearts. Heart attack, a condition in which the heart stops beating properly, and stroke, which affects the arteries leading toward the brain, are the first and fifth top killers of American women.[14] [15] Heart attacks alone strike one in three women a year, meaning that at least one American woman a minute passes away from heart disease. Strokes, linked to high

---

14 "Women's Heart Disease Awareness Study (2012)." Posted February 19, 2013. *American Heart Association:* https://www.goredforwomen.org/about-heart-disease/facts_about_heart_disease_in_women-sub-category/womens-heart-disease-awareness-study-2012/.

15 "Prevention." *American Stroke Association:* http://www.strokeassociation.org/STROKEORG/AboutStroke/About-Stroke_UCM_308529_SubHomePage.jsp (September 19, 2016)

blood pressure and the accumulation of plaque within the circulatory system, aren't just deadly. They are also a leading cause of severe, long-term disability.

Below are warning signs associated with both these illnesses. Should you experience any one of these symptoms—particularly those associated with stroke—please see your doctor immediately. Doing so not only may prevent organ damage but also may save your life.

The American Heart Association's Warning Signs of a Heart Attack[16]

1. **Chest discomfort.** Most heart attacks involve discomfort in the center of the chest that lasts more than a few minutes or goes away and comes back. It can feel like uncomfortable pressure, squeezing, fullness, or pain.

2. **Discomfort in other areas of the upper body.** Symptoms can include pain or discomfort in one or both arms, the back, neck, jaw, or stomach.

3. **Shortness of breath** with or without chest discomfort.

4. **Back pain** with irregular pain in the lower or upper back.

5. **Other signs** may include breaking out in a cold sweat, nausea, or lightheadedness.

"As with men," the same source tells us, "women's most common heart attack symptom is chest pain or discomfort. But women are somewhat more likely than men to experience some of the other common symptoms, particularly shortness of breath, nausea/vomiting and back or jaw pain."[17]

16 "Warning Signs of a Heart Attack." Posted June 2016. *American Heart Association*: http://www.heart.org/HEARTORG/Conditions/HeartAttack/WarningSignsofaHeartAttack/Warning-Signs-of-a-Heart-Attack_UCM_002039_Article.jsp#.V6HvTWVGi-J (August 3, 2016).

17 Ibid.

The American Heart Association's Symptoms of a Stroke[18]

1   Sudden numbness or weakness of the face, arm or leg, especially on one side of the body

2   Sudden confusion or trouble speaking or understanding

3   Sudden trouble seeing or blurred vision in one or both eyes

4   Sudden trouble walking, dizziness, loss of balance, or coordination

5   Sudden severe headache with no known cause

If you find yourself anxious over the possibility of facing one of these struggles, don't be. Make regular wellness visits with your doctor. And remember that through pursuing a healthy diet, exercise, getting rest, managing stress, and eliminating habits like smoking and alcohol consumption, you are investing in the long-term strength and resilience of your heart.

Circle the actions you are taking to prevent spiritual and physical heart disease.

eating nutritious foods	giving up smoking	being active daily
controlling cholesterol	reading God's Word daily	managing blood pressure
thinking clean thoughts	eliminating fried foods	striving for a healthy weight
reducing blood sugar	eliminating sodas	limiting alcohol
controlling diabetes	managing stress	refusing to be a couch potato
getting eight hours of rest nightly	going to God daily for forgiveness	choosing obedience

---

18   "Symptoms of a Stroke." *American Heart Association:* https://www.goredforwomen.org/about-heart-disease/symptoms_of_heart_disease_in_women/symptoms-of-a-stroke/ (August 3, 2016).

Reflections

What do you most want to remember from today's content?

_____

_____

_____

_____

Daily Exercise Prompt

Follow your Cardio TRAIN chart, and don't forget to stretch.

Week Five

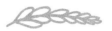

BUILDING STRENGTH

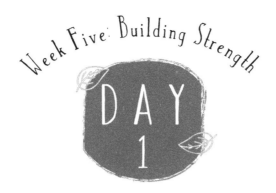

Week Five: Building Strength

DAY 1

GAINING A HEAVENLY PERSPECTIVE

As I sat down to write this week's content, one verse kept coming to mind. Nehemiah 8:10 says, "The joy of the LORD is your strength." As I thought about those words, I realized something important. As we enter this portion of the study that revolves around growing in physical strength, we need to fetch another fruit of the Spirit from our horn of plenty. We also need to do a perspective check. While I could write a hundred pages on physical strength training and its benefits, I know we need spiritual strength even more. Without that, even focused body toning that yields great results will lead us to a sense of emptiness in the long run.

Joy is the character trait or fruit of the Spirit I want us to associate with the following lessons. Joy brings feelings of great happiness, deep delight, and a certainty of success. We first saw the term when I selected green grapes to represent joy. This fruit revitalizes our blood, which feeds muscles. According to one commentator, "The Greek word for *joy* [in reference to the fruit of the

Spirit] is 'chara.' It . . . is a reminder and sign of the way believers [should] view the present in light of God's plan for the future."[1]

Consider these insights into joy. Do you generally view the present in light of God's plan for the future? Why or why not?

_____

_____

_____

In our culture, people tend to think of joy as an elusive thing. One moment we are celebrating a success; the next moment we feel depressed over the regularity of the day-to-day. The future then is something we come to think about in terms of either anticipated personal highs or dreaded lows. And we rarely take time to think that there may be joys before us that far exceed the glory of reaching personal benchmarks. The definition of joy provided by our commentator clarifies that we need to think of joy in a deeper spiritual way than is often considered. As Christians we need to invite the Holy Spirit to make joy a _regular_ part of our life, a thing that is with us constantly and influences the way we view all aspects of life and eternity.

Do you know that with the Spirit's help we can live with an overall sense that everything in our life will work out for the best? It's true! The Bible says that "in all things God works for the good of those who love him, who have been called according to his purpose" (Romans 8:28). And even better, because of our identity in Christ, we can know that our heavenly future will be so fantastic that even the worst days here on this broken planet need not dim our constant joy over the coming prize.

---

1   Thoralf Gilbrant, ed. _The Complete Biblical Library: New Testament Study Bible._ (Springfield, MO: The Complete Biblical Library, 1986), 483-84.

Our Current Physical Bodies Are Temporary

For centuries people have longed to find a cure, a pill, or the fountain of youth to help them stay youthful and healthy. They've sought happiness by trying to turn back the clock. But a harsh truth will always work against the pursuit of such fulfillment: anything we do to improve our bodies now is temporary. All of us from the moment of our birth are in a state of decay and on the fast track to death. The sin that happened in the garden has doomed us to this fate. I don't say this to be morbid. I say it because we can't hang on to youth forever. In fact, trying to do so will only rob us of true, satisfying joy.

Humanity's choice to sin against God is the reason we live with aches and pains and are vulnerable to disease. It's why our lives are sometimes interrupted by funerals. But praise the Lord—we have such a beautiful hope! The hope of humanity is Jesus Christ, who came as the only antidote to the world's sin problem. Jesus stated in John 16:33, "In this world you will have trouble. But take heart! I have overcome the world." Although we are not guaranteed a life free of diseases or afflictions, we have a mighty God who has suffered in our place and has overcome to bring everlasting life to all who will accept Jesus as Lord. Ha-le-lu-yah!

Our Glorious Future

Many don't realize that Christ's followers are promised an amazing and eternal overhaul when we step out of this life and into the next. No passage of Scripture better summarizes what I mean than 2 Corinthians 5:1–4. There Paul writes, "For we know that if the earthly tent we live in [the body] is destroyed, we have a building from God [a new body], an eternal house in heaven, not built by human hands. Meanwhile we groan, longing to be clothed instead with our heavenly dwelling. . . . For while we are in this tent, we groan and are burdened." Did you catch that? Our current bodies will continue to groan no matter what we do, though we should certainly work to maintain them and to minimize wear and tear.

The great news is that restoration is ahead, not just for our souls but also for our bodies. The Bible says that after death, Christians are gifted with new temples, glorious spiritual bodies that are perfect in every way—much like Jesus's body when He walked the earth in His resurrected form. This concept is what Paul meant when he said we have "a building" and "an eternal house in heaven" in contrast to the "tents" we live in here. Paul explains the transformation process this way: "We will all be changed—in a flash, in the twinkling of an eye. . . . Then the saying that is written will come true: 'Death has been swallowed up in victory'" (1 Corinthians 15:51–52, 54). Eugene Peterson, author of the biblical paraphrase *The Message,* sums it up this way: "The corpse that's planted is no beauty, but when it's raised, it's glorious!" (1 Corinthians 15:43–44).

Scripture has so many marvelous things to tell us about the future when we inhabit these new bodies. The book of Revelation is particularly helpful when it says the Lord will create a new heaven and a new earth on which we'll live in those perfected bodies. In that day God will give our planet a makeover similar to ours. He will restore creation to the "very good" state He always intended. There "God's dwelling place [will be] among the people, and he will dwell with them. They will be his people, and God himself will be with them and be their God. He will wipe every tear from their eyes. There will be no more death or mourning or crying or pain, for the old order of things [will pass] away" (Revelation 21:3–4).

Until Then

When you sincerely asked Jesus to be Lord of your life, the Holy Spirit came to live in you, and you received eternal salvation. You are a branch grafted into God's family through Jesus the vine. If you are living in obedience to His Word, the vinedresser is at work in your life daily, preparing your soul for the day when it will fly home with a new body to be with Him forever.

As we ramp up our efforts at fitness this week, know that I want to help you begin to sculpt or maintain the fittest temple possible during the remainder of your earthly stay. But far more important to me is that you know that when this life is over and God is ready to call you home, you will receive an upgraded body that will never know an ache or pain. If you have received Jesus as your Lord and Savior, you have an eternal future with Him, and I can think of nothing more joyous than that!

In the days ahead, use every twinge of discomfort and the sight of every gray hair or wrinkle that greets you in the mirror as a joyful reminder that for the Christian, better days are always ahead.

Reflections

What truths or Scripture verse from today's lesson most spoke to you? Explain.

_____

_____

_____

Daily Exercise Prompt

Today I want you to take a break from your TRAIN routine; instead, put on your walking shoes and go for a nice leisurely walk in a nearby park. As you go, spend some time pondering today's content and asking God to help you live in joyful anticipation of His work in your life and your eternal future with Him. Praise Him for His goodness!

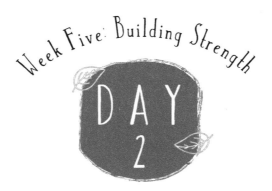

Week Five: Building Strength

DAY 2

FEMALE BODY CHEMISTRY AND
THE ROLE OF FAT AND MUSCLE

Over the next couple of days, we will add specific strength building exercises to the TRAIN regimen you've begun. During my years of teaching fitness, I've learned that some women are hesitant about doing this type of exercise because they don't want to end up looking like a circus strong man. To alleviate any concerns you might have, I am using today's content to cover female body chemistry and to explain the practical benefits of shrinking fat and toning muscle.

Our Shapely Temple

I've previously equated the shape of the average woman with a pear. Sure, some of us are shaped more like rulers or hourglasses or ovals, but the image of the pear resonates with me because it acknowledges the feminine tendency to carry extra curves in the region of our hips and thighs. When I think about the fact that we carry our babies between our hips and then snuggle them across our laps, I gain a deeper appreciation for this truth. Make no mistake—we are divinely designed!

Also helpful to building a healthy respect for the unique qualities God programmed into the feminine form is the realization that our temples carry two kinds of fat, and it's a mistake to think of all fat as a bad thing. The authors of *Lifetime Physical Fitness & Wellness* explain it this way:

> We have "essential" fat and "storage" fat in our bodies. Essential fat is necessary for our daily physiological functions. . . . It is found within tissue such as muscles, nerve cells, bone marrow, intestines, [the] heart, liver and lungs. At least 12% of women's fat is essential fat. Our essential fat also consists of sex-specific fat that is found in the breast tissue, the uterus, and in other sex-related fat deposits.
>
> Storage fat is the fat stored in adipose tissue, mostly just beneath the skin (subcutaneous fat) and around major organs in the body. This fat serves three basic functions. . . . It is (1) an insulator to retain body heat, (2) a[n] energy substrate for metabolism, and (3) padding against physical trauma to the body.[2]

Despite what our culture sometimes indicates, there is no shame in having a well-rounded temple. In fact, you may have noticed that in paintings from earlier eras, beautiful women were always represented with plenty of padding. The ultra-thin look popularized in modern magazines and movies is a departure from historical preferences. It also presents an ideal that is unattainable given most feminine body types and the continuing changes life's stages bring. However, whether we carry many curves or few, all of us can benefit from working to increase our muscle tone and the overall health and strength of our bodies.

---

2   Werner W. K. and Sharon Hoeger, *Lifetime Physical Fitness and Wellness: A Personalized Program* (Belmont, CA: Thomson Wadsworth, 2007), 106.

When most men think about working out, they want to develop bigger and stronger muscles. Women, on the other hand, generally desire to have a strong "toned" looking body in which the outlines of muscles can be noted underneath firm and supple skin. We know intuitively that this—rather than the strong-man look—is attractive and will help us to feel more confident.

Working for us in the pursuit of this toned look is the fact that our bodies are programmed differently than men's. Walters and Byl note this:

> Women's capacity to enlarge their muscles is much more limited than men's. One of the main reasons for this disparity is hormonal; men have 20 to 30 times more testosterone than women do. . . . High levels of testosterone help create a positive environment for building muscle. Another contributing factor is that although women have the same number of muscles that men have, from birth women have fewer individual fibers. These and other factors contribute to women on average having about half (40 to 60 percent) of the upper-body strength and three-quarters (65 to 85 percent) of the lower body strength of their male counterparts.[3]

Benefits of Strength Training

For us women, strength training is generally about changing our overall physique—whatever our underlying shape—from flabby to firm. It's about pursuing muscle tone. Strength training shrinks our fat cells. Werner and Sharon Hoeger explain, "A benefit of strength training, accentuated even more when combined with aerobic exercise, is a ***decrease*** in adipose or fatty tissue around muscle fibers themselves."[4] As our muscles become stronger and enlarge a bit, our fat cells shrink in size. This process will not completely

---

3   Peter Walters and John Byl, *Christian Paths to Health and Wellness.* (Champaign, IL: Human Kinetics, 2013), 109–10.

4   Hoeger and Hoeger, *Lifetime Physical Fitness and Wellness*, 198.

do away with cellulite—that's a fact of female life related to hormones. But it will go a long way in smoothing and firming our bodies. The diagram below will help illustrate this fact about muscle versus fat.

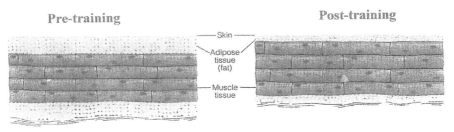

Werner W. K. Hoeger and Sharon Hoeger, *Lifetime Physical Fitness & Wellness*. (Belmont, Calif.: Thomson Wadsworth-Belmont, 2007), 198–99.

Diagram I

The toning process typically leads to our losing inches though not necessarily pounds, since muscle is denser than fat. An added bonus of this process is that it turns our temples into fat-burning machines. Don't miss that! Strength training increases our metabolism so we burn more fat! Peter Walters and John Byl note this:

> Our Resting Metabolic Rate (RMR) is what occurs when our bodies burn calories when we are completely inactive, and is profoundly affected by the amount of lean body mass in our temples. Basically, each pound of muscle burns 30 to 40 calories per day at rest. This makes muscle the most metabolically active substance in the body. (By contrast, a pound of fat burns one to two calories per day.) It follows that a person who gains 5 pounds of muscle will burn 150 to 200 calories per day *doing nothing.*[5]

At this point in our journey, I want to encourage you to hide your bathroom scale for the remainder of our time together. Keep watching what you eat, and don't slow down on your workouts. But keep in mind that the next exercises I'll introduce are meant to tone and build your muscle. That focus may lead

---

5   Walters and Byl, *Christian Paths,* 111.

to a slow-down on the scale in terms of pounds dropped if that is indeed your goal, but we are working to build a healthier you overall. Don't allow a stubborn number to cheat you out of the joy of this part of the journey. Staying the course can lead to big payoffs in the long run.

Reflections

What about today's lesson do you most want to remember?

_____

_____

_____

Daily Exercise Prompt

It's time to get back on track with Cardio TRAIN if you took a break from it yesterday. In addition to your usual routine, try to add at least three simple strength-training ideas that you can find by doing a simple online search for "isometric exercises."[6] Tomorrow I'll explain what that term means and soon will give you a whole list of fun shape-building examples you can start incorporating into your weekly exercise regimen.

---

6   I suggest *prevention.com* or *shapesense.com* as a good place to start.

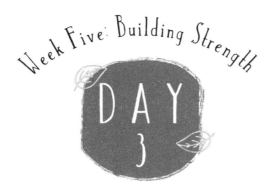

Week Five: Building Strength

DAY 3

FORMS OF STRENGTH TRAINING

I love the visual that Proverbs 31:17 provides us as we dig further into this week's concept: "She sets about her work vigorously; her arms are strong for her tasks." How can we build strong arms and legs for hauling babies, carrying groceries, providing taxi service for our families, playing with our kids, cooking and cleaning our homes, keeping our yards tidy, and just generally keeping up with all life demands? Strength training is the answer, and it appears that the virtuous woman of Proverbs 31 was no stranger to exercise—though I doubt she needed a gym.

Strength training, also referred to as resistance or weight training, is all about lifting various amounts of weight to increase our overall strength and to develop muscle tone. This type of training takes many different forms—including using one's own body weight, various free weights, and machines—to achieve the desired results.[7]

Four Forms

There are four basic types of strength training. The first, which I encouraged you to research and try at the close of our last lesson, is isometric. This is a good place to start. *Iso* means "same," and *metric* means "length." In this type of exercise, we work our muscles without changing the angle of our joints or altering the length of our muscles. Instead, we keep our bodies motionless and simply allow our muscles to hold a contraction. Examples of isometric exercise include sitting against the wall in an imaginary chair and leaning into a doorway as we rest one forearm on either side of the door's frame, or a plank.

The second type of strength training is isotonic. Again, *iso* means "same." *Tonic* means "tension." This type of exercise is all about making a muscle shorten and extend multiple times using a constant load. When we lift five-pound free weights, strap weights to our ankles at the gym, or lift a bar weight with the help of a spotter, we engage in isotonic exercise. The tension (force) we require of the muscles varies while the weight remains the same.

The third type of strength training is known as variable resistance. This type requires us to use differing degrees of force to encourage our muscles to work against constant resistance. For instance, a variable-resistance arm curl requires that the bicep work from the beginning of the movement until its end, increasing its output throughout the motion. Many machines that use pulleys, levers, cams, or barbells with bands offer varying degrees of resistance to facilitate variable-resistance exercises.

---

7   While some forms of strength training are perfectly appropriate activities for children's participation, weightlifting, bodybuilding, or power lifting are not. Too much stress and strain on young muscles may damage growth plates. If your child or grandchild hopes to train with you, lead him or her to exercises like push-ups, Pilates, PiYo, lunges, or squats. Block access to strength-training equipment.

The last type of exercise, frequently used in rehabilitation and physical therapy, is referred to as isokinetic strength training. As you know, *iso* means "same." *Kinetic* refers to motion. In this type of exercise, speed of movement is constant. Machines are made to facilitate this type of workout function, keeping the rate of muscular contraction the same. No matter how hard we may try to push or pull during any given exercise, the speed remains constant. "Athletic trainers and physical therapists often use this type when rehabilitating patients from injury or measuring strength."[8]

Which of the above forms have you tried?

_____

_____

Which sounds most appealing to you?

_____

_____

Benefits

The advantages to adding strength training to our weekly routines are diverse. We covered the first two yesterday.

As you read, place a star beside the statements that most encourage you to make strength training a regular part of your life.

1 **Strength training contributes to building and maintaining a toned, shapely temple.**

---

8   Walters and Byl, *Christian Paths*, 125.

2   **Strength training will help boost fat-burning metabolism.** Note this important insight from *Christian Paths to Health and Wellness*: "Weight training is especially important for people ages 30 to 65, since they lose about half a pound . . . of muscle per year, which is equal to burning approximately 6,387.5 fewer calories [annually]."[9]

3   **Strength training leads to neuromuscular advantages.** Peter Walters and John Byl helpfully comment that "resistance training builds . . . tendon and ligament stability along with skeletal integrity. This enhancement of muscle, bone, and connective tissue has a dramatic effect on lowering one's chance of injury."[10] In other words, the strength of your body is inversely related to your chances of developing a neuromuscular injury. In fact, there is "growing evidence that suggests strengthening the lower back through resistance training can help with lower back pain and in many cases prevent lower back injury."[11] That's a huge help in this sedentary culture in which we live.

4   **Strength training assists in the building of strong bones.** The stretching and lengthening of tendons and ligaments due to resistance training should prevent or delay the onset of osteoporosis. This disease seems to come calling on us ladies during our third and fourth decades, especially after menopause. It is caused by the softening and deterioration of bones as well as a general loss of the mineral density within them. Interestingly, "recent research indicates that resistance training may be just as important if not more important than ingesting adequate levels of calcium [when it comes to fighting the onset of osteoporosis]."[12]

Walters and Byl add this:

---

9   Ibid., 111.
10   Ibid., 113.
11   Ibid..
12   Ibid., 112–13.

Bones consist of hard web-like structures of collagen, calcium, and other minerals; this part of the bone is called the *bone matrix*. The structure of bone matrix leaves gaps in the web, which are filled with bone marrow and blood vessels. Osteoporosis (derived from the Greek words for *bone* and *porous*) is the breakdown of the bone mineral web, making it more vulnerable to compression and shear fractures. This process tends to happen with aging: 55 percent of people over age 50 have low bone density (National Osteoporosis Foundation, 2012). . . . Bone density peaks between ages 20 and 30, but after this climax there is often a faster rate of bone reabsorption [a process by which the calcium within bones is released into the bloodstream], than growth.[13]

5. Strength training improves functional capacity, whether in terms of one's ability to carry heavy objects or to play a better golf game.

6. **Strength training contributes to an overall sense of well-being.** When done regularly, it can improve the quality of sleep, contribute to better glucose control, build healthy heart tissue, and help maintain a healthy state of mind.

Reflections

What about today's lesson do you most wish to remember?

_____

_____

_____

_____

---

13   Ibid., 112.

Daily Exercise Prompt

I sincerely hope that in the days ahead you will allow God to increase your strength and stamina through the types of exercise introduced today. For now, continue with your Cardio TRAIN program, knowing that tomorrow we will look at specific strength-training exercises we can do at home.

If possible, stop by your local gym today for a tour. (No need to join unless you want to do so.) Pay close attention to what strength-training equipment is available, and consider whether a gym membership might prove beneficial as you continue to make fitness a priority.

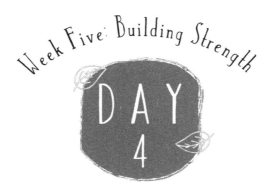

Week Five: Building Strength

DAY 4

STRENGTH TRAINING AT HOME

I hope you were able to tour your local gym yesterday, but gym membership is not required for working to improve tone and increase strength. Instead, we can begin incorporating no-fancy-equipment-needed exercises into our existing TRAIN programs.

Home Strength-Training Ideas

Step one to making strength training a part of your existing routine is to think of whatever you are doing in your cardio plan as a warm-up. This approach will allow the muscles to loosen up and warm before you begin to put them under the demands of strength training. To this I will add that as you begin to incorporate the following ideas into your routine, you will need to start slowly. Muscles new to the activities I'll suggest will need twenty-four to forty-eight hours to rest and rebuild between your first and second workouts. Moreover, if you choose to work out all your muscle groups in one session, working from the largest to the smallest muscles, you won't need to do strength training the following day. In fact, you can do it only once or twice a week and enjoy great results. Another option is to choose to strength train one section of the body at a time, perhaps working leg muscles on day one, core muscles on day two, and the upper body muscles on day three before starting the process all over again the following week. (Again, it's wise to stagger the days on which you strength train.)

The coming suggestions are just a few examples of exercises you can perform easily at home. You will notice I've divided them by which portion of the body they are designed to impact. They are further divided into beginner, intermediate, and advanced levels to accommodate readers of all skill sets and to better equip us to challenge ourselves once we are comfortable with performing the basics.

Today as you read through the instructions given for each of the following exercises, select one exercise under each of the three main subheadings, and walk through the steps. As you do, be aware of the tendency to hold your breath while exercising. A better approach is to breathe steadily, exhaling heavily during the most difficult phases of an exercise. It is important to inhale as we lower into our starting position.

Remember, a *set* is a prescribed number of reps. A *rep* is the number of exercises performed in each set. Example: 1 set of 7 bicep curls= 7 bicep curls performed one right after another, ending in rest.

Lower Body

EXERCISE 1: THE LUNGE (OR SQUAT-SPLITS)

Beginner

1   Stand tall in a doorway with your feet shoulder-width apart. Face forward in a stationary position.

2.   Place your right hand on the doorframe for balance. Then take a big step forward with your left foot so there's about one leg's distance between that foot and your right one. Keep your right leg straight, toes on ground, heel up.

3.   Make certain the top part of your temple remains straight. Hold your shoulders back and tighten your tummy.

4.   Slowly lower your hips until both knees are bent at a ninety-degree angle. You determine how far you wish to lower your right knee, but be sure not to move your left knee over your left toes.

5.   Return to your starting position. This is one rep.

6.   Perform one set of seven reps for each side of your body. To work the opposite side, step out with your right foot.

Intermediate Adjustments

Follow the steps above, but don't allow yourself the support of leaning on a doorway for balance. Complete two sets of ten lunges with each leg.

Advanced Adjustments

Moving away from anything you might be tempted to lean on for balance, perform three sets of fifteen or more reps per leg.

EXERCISE 2: SQUATS

Beginner

1.   Stand with your back to a wall and your feet shoulder-width apart.

2.   Keeping your back against the wall, slowly walk your feet out in front of you as you slide down into a seated position. Your quadriceps, the large muscles on the tops of your legs, should be parallel to the ground. Make sure your knees do not extend past your toes once you are in the seated pose.

3. Remain stationary in this position for ten to fifteen seconds. This is one rep.

4. Slowly stand back up, and then perform one set of four reps.

Intermediate Adjustments

1. Stand with your feet shoulder-width apart while facing a stationary object like a kitchen island.

2. Place both palms flat against the top of the stationary object at arm's length as you lower yourself into a squat much like before, and hold it for ten to fifteen seconds. Quadriceps should be parallel to the floor, the back straight, and the abdomen muscles tight.

3. Slowly stand up straight. This is one rep.

4. Perform one set of seven to ten reps.

Advanced Adjustments

1. Stand clear of objects, and place your feet shoulder-width apart.

2. Squat, unsupported, until your quads are parallel to the floor.
   Clasp your hands in front of you for balance. (Your chest may be at a 45-degree angle.) Hold it for ten to fifteen seconds.

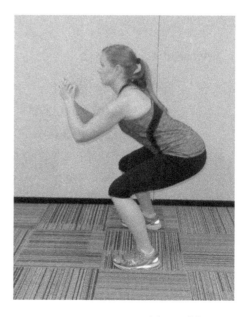

3. Slowly stand up straight. This completes one rep.

4. Perform two sets of ten to fifteen reps or more.

Advanced Squat

EXERCISE 3: THREE-STAGE TOE RAISES

Beginner

1. Grab a timer, and set it for fifteen seconds. Stand up straight and face forward while holding on to a kitchen island or desk. Your feet should be shoulder-width apart, and your toes should point forward.

2. Slowly raise your body weight, balancing on your toes as if preparing to tiptoe across the room. Keep your back and shoulders straight. The chin should be parallel to the floor.

3. Lower your body so your feet are once again flat on the floor, and repeat steps 2 and 3 until fifteen seconds have passed.

4. Reset the timer for another fifteen seconds. This time, point your toes outward at about a 45-degree angle so your heels are close together.

5. Slowly raise your body weight as before.

6. Lower your body and repeat steps 5 and 6 until fifteen seconds have passed.

7. Reset the timer for another fifteen seconds. Now point your toes toward each other.

8. Slowly raise your body weight as before.

9. Perform actions 7 and 8 continuously for fifteen seconds.

Intermediate Adjustments

Perform the above exercises for twenty seconds each. Allow a twenty-second rest period in between working through each of the three main positions.

Advanced Adjustments

Perform the above exercises for thirty seconds each. Allow a twenty-second rest period in between working through each of the three main positions.

Core or Middle Body

EXERCISE 1: REVERSE CRUNCH

Beginner

1. Lie flat on your back with your arms resting against your sides and your hands flat on the floor. Raise your legs so it would appear from the side that you are sitting in a chair, with the ground being the chairback.

2. Using the muscles in your mid-section and not your hands, pull both knees toward your chest, and then return to the starting position. This is one rep.

3. Perform one set of five to seven reps.

Intermediate Adjustments

Perform two sets of ten to twelve reps, using the above directions.

Advanced Adjustments

Perform three sets of twelve reps, using the above directions. This time, pull both knees all the way to your chest, and then extend your heels straight up toward the ceiling.

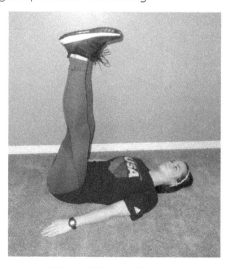

Advanced Reverse Crunch

EXERCISE 2: PILATES PLANK

(A plank is a type of exercise used in Pilate training and is available in DVD form. Pilate moves are excellent for strengthening your core.)

Beginner

1. Situate your body face down in a modified push-up position, which is great for women. With your hands and knees on the floor, bend your knees so the soles of your feet face the ceiling. Your palms should rest on the floor directly under your shoulders. The rest of your body should be aligned straight from your knees to your head at a 45-degree angle.

2. Using your arms and abdominal muscles, hold this position for ten to fifteen seconds. This is one set.

3. Complete two sets, and don't forget to rest for fifteen seconds between them.

Intermediate Adjustments

1. Situate yourself in a more traditional push-up pose. Straighten out your legs behind you so only your hands and toes are on the floor. Keep your back and body straight.

2. Hold that position for fifteen to twenty seconds. This is one set.

3. Perform three or more sets. Rest for twenty seconds between sets.

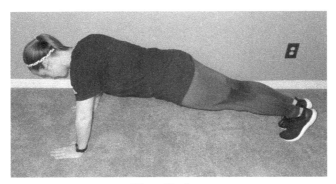

Pilates Plank

Advanced Adjustments

1. Follow the instructions given for the intermediate approach to the Pilates plank.

2. Hold this position for thirty to forty-five seconds. This is one set.

3. Perform two or three sets. Rest for thirty seconds between sets.

EXERCISE 3: PILATES AND PIYO

Find Pilates or PiYo exercises you would like to use to work on your core. You can find exercise videos online or on DVD.

Upper Body

EXERCISE 1: WALL PUSH-UPS

Beginner

1. Stand an arm's length from a wall, facing it with your feet flat on the floor.

2. Place your palms flat against the wall at the same level as your shoulders and slightly wider than shoulder-width.

3. Slowly bend your elbows, and lower the weight of your body until you can touch your forehead to the wall.

4. Gently push yourself back to the starting position, keeping your body straight throughout this movement. This is one rep.

5. Perform two sets of seven reps.

Intermediate Adjustments

1. Stand an arm's length from a kitchen island or desk. Rest your palms against its surface. Your feet should be flat on the floor.

2. Slowly lower your chest to the immovable object and back up to your starting position. Keep your knees slightly bent throughout this movement. This is one rep.

3. Perform two sets of ten reps. Don't forget to breathe.

Advanced Adjustments

1. Do a girls' push-up. Lie down, palms on the floor and slightly wider apart than shoulder-width. Bend your knees at a 45-degree angle with the bottoms of your feet facing the ceiling. Push up to where your upper torso is at a 45-degree angle and your stomach stays close to the floor.

2. Perform two sets of fifteen reps.

EXERCISE 2: BICEP CURLS

Beginner

1. Stand upright with your arms resting by your sides. Open your hands so your palms face your body.

2. Bend at the elbow, and slowly raise thumbs up to your shoulders and lower. This is one rep.

3. Complete three sets of ten reps.

Intermediate Adjustments

1. Complete the bicep curl, but rather than having empty hands, hold a half-filled water bottle in each. (Bottles may be filled with water or sand.)

2. Perform three sets of twenty reps.

Advanced Adjustments

1. Complete the bicep curl, this time holding a full water bottle in each hand.

2. Perform three sets of twelve to fifteen reps. Give yourself twenty seconds' rest between each set.

EXERCISE 3: TRICEPS CURLS

Beginner

1. Stand upright with your hands by your sides, palms facing your body.

2. Slowly extend your arms out in front of your body, parallel to the floor.

3. Bend your arms up and toward your body until your thumbs touch your shoulders.

4. Extend your arms straight again. This is one rep.

5. Perform three sets of seven reps.

Intermediate Adjustments

1. Stand upright with your arms and hands extended, reaching toward the ceiling. In each hand, hold a half-filled water bottle.

2. Bend your arms until your elbows face the ceiling and your hands are behind your back.

3. Slowly raise your hands up to the ceiling from that position, and then lower them back down. This is one rep.

4. Perform three sets of ten to fifteen reps.

Advanced Adjustments

1. Follow the intermediate instructions above, this time using full water bottles.

2. Complete three sets of twenty reps.

Incorporating Strength Training into an Existing TRAIN Chart

Before you begin adding to the TRAIN chart you've begun, take time to think through which exercises you want to do on an ongoing basis. Then fill out the TRAIN-for-strength information I've included below. Remember—I do not want you to strength-train more than three days a week, and I encourage you to think carefully about which section(s) of your body to train on which day. Additional insights are included throughout.

My Strong Temple Strength Train

Type of Exercises

(Select a variety of lower, core, and upper-body activities to incorporate into your weekly workout regimen. Unless you already have a strength-training system in place, choose from those ideas I've included above to keep things simple. For instance, you may select a combination of isotonic and isokinetic exercises that use only your body weight. Beginners may want to do lunges and squats for **lower** body, planks for the **core** area, and wall push-ups for **upper** body in that **muscle group order**.)

Race the Clock

(Think about how much time you will spend on strength training in a session. I suggest allowing for three to five minutes of strength-training exercises in the first week you do them.)

A-*Accountability person*

(The person you will inform about your workout regimen so that he or she can keep you on track. In my case, for instance, I'd tell my neighbor Betty about the changes I'm making. She works out with me.)

Intensity

(Record how many sets and reps you'll do of each exercise. (Add amount of weight when you begin to use weights.) In the beginning your routine may look something like this: Lunges and squats = one set of seven reps; plank = two sets with fifteen seconds' rest between sets; push-ups = two sets of seven reps).

Number of Days

(Assign specific activities to specific days; for instance, you may choose to strength-train on only Tuesdays and Thursdays after cardio.)

Now that you have your basic information, revisit the Cardio TRAIN you made earlier. Using what you've learned today and working up to a 150-minute-a-week overall exercising goal, weave these strength-training exercises into your plan.

I sincerely hope you'll try the home strength-training ideas suggested today. But I am equally eager that you work with machines or free weights at the local gym if that is more appealing to you. A personal trainer can help you develop a plan to get you on the fast track to achieving tone. How you go about strengthening your body is up to you.

There are two more points I want to make before we close today. In the days ahead as you begin to work out more rigorously, you are bound to get a little sore if such activity is new for you. If that's the case, remember that rest is your friend. Stretch those warm muscles after exercising, and take a break when you need to. Keep Psalm 28:7–8 in mind: "The LORD is my strength and my shield; my heart trusts in him, and he helps me. My heart leaps for joy, with my song I praise him. The LORD is the strength of his people."

Reflections

Which of the exercises presented in today's content are you most likely to use regularly?

_____

_____

_____

_____

Daily Exercise Prompt

If you haven't done so already, put the above suggestions into practice. Run in place for three minutes as a quick warm-up. Then perform the beginner exercises introduced today, taking a rest of about thirty seconds between each one. When you're finished, do some of the stretches presented in Appendix B as a cool down. And remember—your muscles will need twenty-four to forty-eight hours to rest and rebuild.

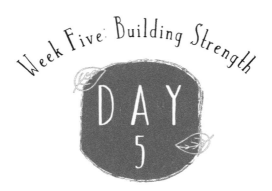

DAY 5

IMPROVING FLEXIBILITY

Spiritual Flexibility

Before we close out this week with a discussion of physical flexibility, I want to talk about the need for spiritual elasticity. As sure as we must remain connected to Jesus, our vine, we must take care not to allow our dedication to God to become stagnant or tradition-based. Instead, our relationship with Him should be dynamic and always growing. This is accomplished as we study His Word regularly, pray without ceasing, live in obedience, and work to spread His love to others. All these activities are like spiritual stretches that keep us fit for the tasks ahead.

Basing your response on that last paragraph, how faithfully are you stretching your temple spiritually?

Very faithfully   Somewhat faithfully   Not at all

What if anything needs to change regarding your approach to spiritual flexibility?

_____

_____

_____

The apostle Paul provides a wonderful example for us regarding this topic. In 1 Corinthians 9 he explains that he dedicated himself to the mission of spreading the good news of Christ like a "runner" in "strict training." He made himself a servant to everyone so he could gain increasing opportunities to lead more people to place faith in Jesus. To reach Jews, he lived as a Jew. To reach Gentiles, he lived as a Gentile. Everything this man did was geared toward advancing the gospel, toward effectively spreading the good news of Jesus and what He came to do. In other words, Paul sought to remain spiritually flexible. He kept his relationship with Jesus and his interactions with others in a constant state of growth so he could make the most of each opportunity God provided.

Paul is an excellent role model for us when it comes to spiritual things. We too should run after Christ like Olympians in a dash, constantly on the lookout for ways to encourage others to invite Jesus to be their Savior. If the last time you shared the gospel with someone seems like a dim memory, it is past time to get serious about spiritual fitness. (And if you aren't certain what I mean by sharing the gospel, please pause to read Appendix A.)

Write the names of three people with whom you can share the good news of salvation through faith in Christ.

1

2

3

Which of the following will you do to help someone hear the good news of Jesus today?

___ Tell a coworker about the Lord

___ Talk to my kids about their need for salvation

___ Send an e-mail or letter to a friend who needs to know Jesus

___ Adopt a missionary through a gospel-based mission organization

Physical Flexibility

Since the start of our time together, I've encouraged you to wrap up each exercise session with stretching. Static stretching refers to elongating or bending a muscle or group of muscles. It involves holding a body part stationary for ten to sixty seconds to lengthen that muscle so it will become more flexible and less prone to stiffness.

Stretching not only provides a wonderful cool down but also helps prevent injuries and lower back pain. A study conducted by H. A. DeVries and G. M. Adams "has discovered that moderate stretching relieves stress and is more effective than prescription medications for reducing muscular tension."[14] In the book *Science of Flexibility*, M. J. Alter adds that stretching leads to a "union of mind and body, self-discipline and self-knowledge, body fitness, posture, and symmetry, relief of muscle cramps and soreness, enjoyment and pleasure, and enhanced sleep."[15] This author later notes, "Regular stretching seems to have a positive effect on performance, particularly if stretching follows the activity."[16] And this practice has one more important benefit: stretching can help compensate for a reduction in natural collagen. At around age thirty, women start to lose this primary connective protein that enables their bodies to stay flexible and supple. This means stretching is an anti-aging tool!

---

14 H. A. DeVries and G. M. Adams, *American Journal of Physical Medicine*, 1972, 51, in Walters and Byl, *Christian Paths*, 146.

15 M J. Alter, *Science of Flexibility* (Champaign, IL: Human Kinetics, 2004), 8–14.

16 Ibid.

"Flexibility," Walters and Byl add, "is the ability of a joint or group of joints to move freely through a full range of motion."[17] Being flexible allows us the freedom to move our bodies in various directions without pain. This "is important for daily activities in general as well as sports performance. Without regular stretching, . . . muscles will tighten and the range of motion in . . . joints will decrease [with] age. This can put a damper on active lifestyles and even hinder day-to-day activities. Things like getting dressed or reaching for something can become extremely difficult without being flexible."[18] In other words, without working to maintain flexibility, we'll quickly become more prone to injury.

The American College of Sports Medicine (2011) suggests we stretch "daily to achieve greater gains."[19] Though the practice is a natural follow-up to an exercise session, anytime of the day or night is a good time to stretch—if muscles are already a bit warm. Even television time after a hot bath provides excellent opportunities for retaining flexibility.

I hope you have been stretching those warmed-up muscles after your cardio and strength- training sessions each week. The goal today is to add your favorite stretches to your existing TRAIN routine. To begin, fill out this prescription for flexibility TRAINing. Specific exercises are listed in Appendix B.

MY BASIC FLEXIBILITY TRAINING PRESCRIPTION

I plan to implement these *types* of flexibility exercise: _____, _____, _____, *racing the clock* by holding each stretch for ten to sixty seconds, a total of _____ minutes. I will ask _____

---

17   Walters and Byl, *Christian Paths*, 138.

18   J. Mueller and N. Nicholas, "Reference Guide to Stretching: An In-depth Look at Flexibility." *SparkPeople*: http://www.sparkpeople.com/reource/fitness_articles.asp?id=10344 p. 1 (August 3, 2011).

19   Ibid., 1.

to partner with me for *accountability*. I will faithfully perform each stretch for one to two sets with three to five reps to monitor the *intensity* of my workout, adjusting as needed. The *number of days* I will work out each week is _____.

If you feel your current chart is looking crowded, know that it's okay to begin again on a fresh piece of construction paper or cardstock. (It may be fun to use a neon or pastel-colored sheet this time.) Spreadsheets are fun also! Incorporate these stretches into the TRAIN chart on the following page. This comprehensive template may help you simplify and incorporate your TRAINs.

Reflections

What about today's content do you most wish to remember?

_____

_____

_____

Daily Exercise Prompt

Turn on some praise music, and work through your comprehensive TRAIN.

COMPREHENSIVE TRAIN CHART

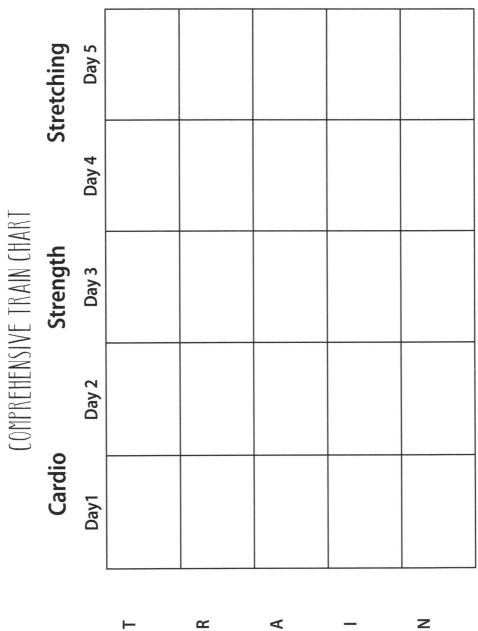

	Cardio		Strength		Stretching
	Day1	Day 2	Day 3	Day 4	Day 5
T					
R					
A					
I					
N					

Chart N

Week Six

OVERCOMING BARRIERS
TO WELLNESS

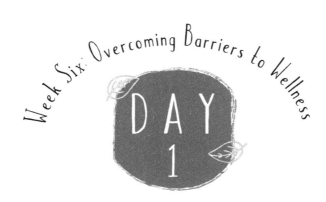

Week Six: Overcoming Barriers to Wellness

DAY 1

PREVENTING A FEAR OF CANCER

You now have the tools you need to eat well, to exercise correctly, and to become your physical best. This week as we wrap up our study, I want to talk about a few barriers to wellness: fear of illness, the pull of addiction, a lack of stress management, and a lack of sleep. As we move through each of these topics, I will advise on how to overcome them. And before the week is over, we'll take a good, long look at the importance of continuously abiding in Christ no matter what we face. He is so very good!

Today we will focus on the importance of relying on Jesus when considering the possibility of developing a debilitating sickness, particularly cancer. In the United Sates a female has a one-in-three chance of developing cancer at some point within her lifetime.[1] According to the U.S. National Cancer Institute, the risk of dying from cancer is one in five.[2] With statistics like that

---

1   "Lifetime Risk of Developing or Dying from Cancer." Posted March 23, 2016. *American Cancer Society:* http://www.cancer.org/cancer/cancerbasics/lifetime-probability-of-developing-or-dying-from-cancer (August 16, 2016).

2   Ibid.

working against us, it makes sense that many live in terror of developing this disease.

Education

The first step to easing a dread of cancer is education. We need to understand the enemy. Consider these basics provided by the American Cancer Society:

> Each of us has around 100 trillion cells in our bodies that reproduce themselves in orderly ways. Under normal conditions these cells continue to grow and reproduce many times. Sometimes our cell growth is disrupted and mutant cells can develop. Some of these cells might grow uncontrollably and abnormally, forming a mass of tissue called a tumor, which can be either benign or malignant. Benign tumors do not invade other tissues. Although they can interfere with normal bodily functions, they rarely cause death. A malignant tumor is a cancer. More than 100 types of cancer can develop in any tissue or organ of the human body. It can start any place in the body.[3]

Cancer is identified by the location in which it starts. Left unchecked, cancer cells can spread to other parts of the body in a process called *metastasis*. Some cancers grow slowly, and some move quickly. Their progress is cataloged under four stages ranging from one to four. Cancer in stages one and two has not spread much. In stages three and four, the cancer has spread and is sometimes fatal. One reason doctors categorize cancer into these stages is so they can determine what form of treatment is best: surgery, chemotherapy, radiation, or—in some advanced cases—hospice care.

Many risk factors contribute to a person's likelihood of developing this disease in some part of the body. We've already addressed several as we've

---

3   "What Is Cancer?" Posted December 8, 2015. *American Cancer Society:*
     http://www.cancer.org/cancer/cancerbasics/what-is-cancer (August 16, 2016).

touched on the need to exercise, eliminate fatty foods, and avoid ingesting high quantities of alcohol or using tobacco products. Other risks are beyond our sphere of control, especially those that are genetic (inherited).

The wisest course of action, then, is to visit our doctors regularly and to keep a close eye on our bodies so even if cancer does develop, we can begin treating it in its earliest stages. This is the thinking behind the modern push for monthly self-breast examinations and annual pap smears and mammograms.

The following list catalogs some of the many signs and symptoms of cancer. Should you experience one or more of the following, do not panic—not every abnormality leads to a cancer diagnosis. Just schedule a visit with your physician as soon as you can.

> unexplained weight loss
>
> fatigue that does not get better with rest
>
> lingering fever
>
> a pain that does not go away
>
> skin changes, like increased darkness or redness (make sure to wear your sunblock!)
>
> sores that will not heal
>
> changes in bowel habits or bladder functions
>
> white patches inside the mouth or white spots on the tongue
>
> nagging cough or hoarseness
>
> indigestion or trouble swallowing
>
> recent changes in a wart or mole
>
> unusual bleeding or discharge
>
> thickening in the breast or other parts of the body.[4]

---

4   "Signs and Symptoms of Cancer." Posted August 11, 2014. *American Cancer Society:* *http://www.cancer.org/cancer/cancerbasics/signs-and-symptoms-of-cancer* (August 16, 2016).

Given what you've learned in this section, do you need to make an
appointment with your primary care doctor? Explain your answer.

_____

_____

_____

Success Stories

Over the years I've come to believe that one of the most helpful tools the
Lord gives us to help us live without a fear of this particular illness is all the
wonderful stories of people who survived a cancer scare. For instance, in early
2015 one of my students developed cancer. After undergoing surgery and
radiation treatments, she was declared to be in remission and has remained
so for eighteen months. Another student survived testicular cancer. After
enduring rounds of treatment and enlisting much prayer from family and
church members, he too is now in remission. And one more student shared
that while her mother had been diagnosed with breast cancer in July 2007
and underwent a lumpectomy and chemo, she is now going into her ninth
year of remission!

My own brush with this dreaded disease began when I noticed a small lump
on my body. This led me to make an appointment with our family physician,
who told me, "I am sending you to a specialist to find out what this growth is."

I'm happy to say I remained calm at this bad news. But after undergoing a
series of tests, I soon found myself standing outside the cancer section of
the hospital. It was then, as I stood with my hand in my husband's, that
thoughts of my mortality threatened to overwhelm me. I began to cry: I felt
God still had a lot for me to do. I didn't want to leave my husband, children,
and grandchildren without a wife, mom, and Gramsie. Thankfully, that same
day I went to the Lord in earnest prayer over the matter and got a handle on
my emotions.

Several biopsies later, the physicians were still uncertain whether the growth was benign or malignant. I underwent surgery so they could remove the entire lump and examine it more closely. Praise God, I am so happy to report those latter test results all came back negative! I was cancer free.

Stories like these are so important to keep in mind. Cancer is not always a death sentence, and we should not think of it as such. Many times it is only a hurdle in our journey, one that makes us stronger and can even give others—doctors, nurses, friends—the chance to hear about our love for Jesus and our hope of an eternity better than anything we know on earth.

Remember Who Is in Charge

The last tool I want to bring up as a weapon against fear is one that came to me as I read Psalm 139:16: "All the days ordained for me were written in your book before one of them came to be." God grants each of us a certain number of days. Whether illness, an injury, or other causes take us out of the game, all of us will eventually expire. Cancer or disease, then, is perhaps rightly thought of as just one of the many vehicles that could drive us home. As Christians, we need not fear death.

I want to pause for a moment to grab another fruit—gentleness—from our horn of plenty (p. 37). Gentleness is a fruit of the Spirit, and you may remember that I selected red grapes and blueberries to represent it. These contain a lot of antioxidants, which are known to house cancer-fighting agents—appropriate, isn't it?

Interestingly, the Greek word *praus* or *prautes* can mean "gentle."[5] Commentator Thoralf Gilbrant notes that when a person has the character trait of gentleness, she will have "a gentle disposition" that will allow her to meet "unhappy circumstances without hostility."[6] Gentleness " is that attitude of spirit by which

---

5   Spiros Zodhiates and Warren Patrick Baker, eds., *Hebrew-Greek Key Word Study Bible NIV*. New Testament Lexical Aids. (Chattanooga, TN: AMG Publishers, 1996), 1665.

6   Thoralf Gilbrant, ed., *The Complete Biblical Library: New Testament Study Bible*. (Springfield, MO: The Complete Biblical Library, 1986), 280.

we accept God's dealings as good and do not dispute or resist."[7] I bring this up because each of us, as daughters of God through faith in His Son, Jesus, will sometimes face bad news—possibly including life-changing medical diagnoses. But rather than growing angry, despairing over negative reports, or even blaming God as if He were out to get us, we must approach our mighty Helper and Healer with gentleness and gratitude. We must remember that He is near, He is good, and He is love. We can face *anything* with His help.

Should fear threaten to steal your joy, hang on to this passage:

> Rejoice in the Lord always. I will say it again: Rejoice! Let your gentleness be evident to all. The Lord is near. Do not be anxious about anything, but in every situation, by prayer and petition, with thanksgiving, present your requests to God. And the peace of God, which transcends all understanding, will guard your hearts and your minds in Christ Jesus.
>
> Finally, brothers and sisters, whatever is true, whatever is noble, whatever is right, whatever is pure, whatever is lovely, whatever is admirable—if anything is excellent or praiseworthy—think about such things. Whatever you have learned or received or heard from me, or seen in me—put it into practice. And the God of peace will be with you. (Philippians 4:4–9)

Reflections

What from today's material most spoke to you?

_____

[Daily Exercise Prompt]
Work through all your Cardio TRAIN.

---

7   Zodhiates and Baker, *Hebrew-Greek Key Word Study Bible NIV*, 1665.

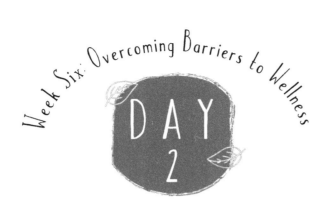

Week Six: Overcoming Barriers to Wellness

DAY 2

FIGHTING ADDICTIONS

According to the book *Lifetime Physical Fitness & Wellness*, "Psychotherapists have described addiction as a problem of imbalance or unease within the body and mind. . . . Almost anything can be addicting. . . . The most serious form is chemical dependency on drugs such as tobacco, alcohol, cocaine, methamphetamine, MDMA (Ecstasy), heroin, marijuana, or prescription drugs. Less serious are addictions to work, coffee, shopping, and even exercise."[8] Any of these dependencies can become barriers between an addict and good health. And any of these dependencies can represent very real struggles for Christians.

Perhaps you saw the title of today's lesson and thought, *I don't have any addictions,* or maybe, *So-and-so needs to read this!* But considering the above definition, it's wise for each of us to do a thorough self-evaluation.

---

8   Werner W.K. and Sharon Hoeger, *Lifetime Physical Fitness and Wellness: A Personalized Program.* (Belmont, CA: Thomson Wadsworth, 2007), 386.

Might you be addicted to any of the following? Circle those that apply.

- hoarding • habitual shopping • eating too much or too little
- smoking • obsessing • social media • prescription drug abuse
- technological devices • chemical dependence • alcohol abuse
- overwork • sleeping pill dependency • over-exercising • other:

Step One

If you drew a circle or two in that last activity, don't berate yourself. Instead, rejoice—because you've taken an important step toward breaking free of the problem. You've admitted there is an issue, and you've courageously given it a name.

> **_Take a moment to read this helpful truth from 1 Corinthians 10:13 aloud:_**

> No temptation has overtaken you except what is common to mankind. And God is faithful; he will not let you be tempted beyond what you can bear. But when you are tempted, he will also provide a way out so that you can endure it.

Don't miss the hope of this verse. No matter your struggle, whether it's overspending or overindulging, what you face is a common part of living in a fallen world. But our God is faithful! He knows what most tempts you, and He does provide help.

God sends help from the "fruit of the Spirit, _enkrateia_. This Greek word for _self-control_ will help us 'overcome' an assortment of addictions. The fruit is seen as the result of the indwelling of the Spirit, not primarily of the willpower of humans. _Enkrateia_ is self-control, abstinence from something, power or control over oneself.' Remember from the 'classical Greek, self-control was a sign of human freedom: one is truly free if he/she could control his [her passions].'"[9] Allow the Holy Spirit to fill you with power and control over any addiction you are facing.

Step Two

The key to overcoming an addiction or even a bad habit is to seek support. Yes, speaking to our usual accountability partners about our hang-ups can be helpful, but the truth is that most addicts and long-time strugglers benefit most from professional medical help. I strongly advise anyone fighting a battle like those we're discussing to seek out the assistance of a doctor or a licensed Christian counselor and to join a supportive recovery group like Celebrate Recovery or Alcoholics Anonymous. In cases where detox is recommended by a physician or counselor, it's important that the addict—and her network of supporters—take the process seriously. Addicts benefit most from committing to a full regimen of treatment and reprogramming.

The great news is that help for fighting any kind of addiction or obsession is available, but we must reach for it.

Step Three

For Christians, the final step toward defeating an addiction of any kind involves deepening our relationship with God, our vinedresser, and developing our understanding of His will for us by spending time in prayer, studying and meditating on His Word, and becoming more sensitive to the leading of the Holy Spirit.

1   First, we need to recognize that we are no longer our own. We answer to the Lord and by our actions can set ourselves up for blessings or curses.

---

9   Gilbrant, *The Complete Biblical Library*, 212-13.

- You were bought at a price. Therefore honor God with your bodies. (1 Corinthians 6:20)

- Do not be deceived: God cannot be mocked. A man reaps what he sows. Whoever sows to please their flesh, from the flesh will reap destruction; whoever sows to please the Spirit, from the Spirit will reap eternal life. (Galatians 6:7–9)

- See, I am setting before you today a blessing and a curse—the blessing if you obey the commands of the LORD your God that I am giving you today; the curse if you disobey the commands of the LORD your God and turn from the way that I command you today by following other gods. (Deuteronomy 11:26-28)

2. Second, we must remember that making choices that honor God is an act of worship that leads to clarity of thought and thus to wiser actions in the future.

- You were taught, with regard to your former way of life, to put off your old self, which is being corrupted by its deceitful desires; to be made new in the attitude of your minds; and to put on the new self, created to be like God in true righteousness and holiness. (Ephesians 4:22-24)
  Therefore, I urge you, brothers and sisters, in view of God's mercy, to offer your bodies as a living sacrifice, holy and pleasing to God—this is your true and proper worship. Do not conform to the pattern of this world, but be transformed by the renewing of your mind. Then you will be able to test and approve what God's will is—his good, pleasing and perfect will. (Romans 12:1-2)

3. Third, we must remember that rather than taking us to heaven immediately when we accept Jesus as Savior, the Lord leaves us on earth to join Him in the work of pointing others to Jesus. There is much purposeful work for each of us to do. Who has time for addiction to anything but Christ?

- You are . . . God's special possession, that you may declare the praises of him who called you out of darkness into his wonderful light. (1 Peter 2:9)

- "Therefore go and make disciples of all nations, baptizing them in the name of the Father and of the Son and of the Holy Spirit, and teaching them to obey everything I have commanded you. And surely I am with you always, to the very end of the age." Matthew 28:19–20)

- We are God's handiwork, created in Christ Jesus to do good works, which God prepared in advance for us to do. (Ephesians 2:10)

Dear sister, if you are struggling with an addiction, it's time to ask the Lord's help in fighting it. You've admitted your struggle. Now seek the professional and Christian assistance you need, and learn to think of yourself in light of your identity as a beloved daughter of God. I pray the Lord will set you gloriously and forever free!

Reflections

What concepts or verses from today's material do you most wish to remember or share?

_____

_____

[Daily Exercise Prompt]
Work through all your TRAIN chart today.

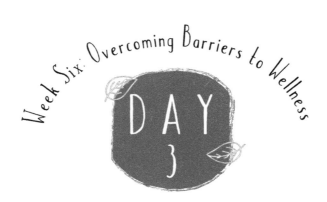

Week Six: Overcoming Barriers to Wellness

DAY 3

MANAGING STRESS

"Stress," explain Werner and Sharon Hoeger, "is the mental, emotional, and physiological response of the body to any situation that is new, threatening, frightening, or exciting."[10] It exists in two forms. The first form is *eustress*, which is quite positive. It is the kind of healthy anticipation and drive we feel when we prepare to get married or celebrate a job promotion. Often our quality of performance increases when we are under this type of stress. The other form, *distress*, places us in a negative emotional state that can lead to unpleasant physical consequences. It often shows up in our life when work is hectic, when our schedules are too busy, or when we face ongoing family or financial concerns that we simply can't resolve. Frankly, being under this kind of stress can feel as if we are engaged in war. If wellness is our goal, it's time we learned how to manage the chaos.

---

10   Werner and Hoeger, *Lifetime Physical Fitness and Wellness*, 357.

What situations in your life lead to feelings of distress?

• tardiness • car troubles • missing items • too much stuff
• sick children • financial concerns • medical issues • marriage troubles
• over-commitment • disrespectful children • the death of a loved one
• raising children with special needs • work concerns • other:

Which of the following stress-management tools have you tried? Check all that apply.

praying

talking my troubles out on family and friends

performing cardio exercise

writing in a journal

doing strength training

singing

listening to praise-and-worship music

learning deep-breathing methods

dancing

making lists

taking naps

stretching

keeping detailed schedules

playing a musical instrument

taking bubble baths

reading

eating well

getting plenty of sleep

pursuing a hobby

seeking alone time

receiving professional counseling

fellowshipping with other Christians

reading the Bible daily

Lawrence H. Roe Jr., a family friend and licensed medical physician, says that managing stress is best approached through a combination of coping mechanisms. He suggests "regular visits with your doctor, exercise, eating well, getting nightly rest, abstaining from substances, and praying regularly" as tools for overcoming it.

> **With that combination approach to stress management in mind, write yourself a multi-step anti-stress prescription. Feel free to incorporate suggestions from above, and make sure that at least one of your steps focuses on strengthening your relationship with God.**

_____

_____

_____

Here's mine: *I manage stress by turning immediately to the Lord for wisdom, guidance, and peace. I listen to Christian praise-and-worship music, talk to my prayer warriors for support, exercise, eat healthily, and get enough rest.*

Choosing Peace

Left unmanaged, stress can begin to affect heart and breathing rates. It can lead to headaches, back pain, sweaty palms, and nausea. And over time it can lead to depression. In fact, stress can become so debilitating that I don't want to close our discussion of it without sharing what I believe to be *the* antidote to the problem. It's the fix we need if we are to overcome the crippling effects of stress once and for all.

We need the gift of spiritual peace.

Earlier on our horn of plenty, I listed peace among the spiritual fruits and represented it with the banana. The banana is one of the central ingredients of the well-known BRAT diet, which doctors use to get an upset stomach and out-of-whack digestive system back on track. Thus, it seems an appropriate choice for conveying the kind of calm intended in the Galatians passage. Peace can get our swirling emotions back under control. "*Eirene* is the Greek word for 'peace.' [It] means [to] live in harmony and tranquility. Peace is also associated with a peaceful attitude."[11] This is just what we need to avoid becoming shipwrecked by life's many stressors.

In sharing my own anti-stress prescription, I admitted that I do sometimes struggle with stress—even though I have firsthand experience with this secret weapon's power against it. The great news is that *I am learning* to request peace on an ongoing basis, and it is *slowly* becoming my default reaction when life gets rocky. The trend began during a very challenging season in which our gracious vinedresser provided peace for me when I desperately needed it. With the help of the Holy Spirit at work within me, I saw for myself the truth of Isaiah 26:3—"You [God] will keep in perfect peace those whose minds are steadfast, because they trust in you."

About the time I received the difficult medical reports I discussed in day one of this week, my oldest daughter faced a health crisis of her own. She was scheduled for a difficult female surgery in a city a thousand miles away from my loving care, and it would be up to her young husband to be her total caregiver. While I knew my son-in-law adored my daughter and would do his best for her, my heart grieved. I thought of all the things she would have to endure that only another woman could understand. I felt as if I were letting her down, but I knew there was no way I could leave my job and responsibilities to provide nursing assistance that was already covered. So I decided to lean hard on the Lord and His promises. I started praying every hour and clung especially hard to 1 Peter 5:7, which says, "Cast all your anxiety on him because he cares for you."

Missionary J. Oswald Sanders once wisely stated, "Peace isn't the absence of trouble but the presence of God in the midst of trouble. The blessing of true peace gives us the ability to make it through anything, knowing that God sees our progress report and is using every problem to teach us. And in turn, we can be a blessing by comforting and teaching others."[12] With that in mind,

---

11   Gilbrant, *The Complete Biblical Library*, 280–82.

12   Mari Lee Parish, *Count Your Blessings: Inspiration from the Beloved Hymn* (Uhrichsville, OH: Barbour Publishing, 2012), 35.

I ramped up my prayers from every hour to turning every single moment of anxiety into an opportunity to pray. I gave concerns to the Lord as soon as they popped into my head and asked Him to shape and teach me even during my sadness and worry.

Slowly I noticed an amazing change. It wasn't long until I realized that rather than focusing on my own struggles, I found myself keeping my ears attuned to hear the needs of others. While I couldn't do anything for my daughter beyond calling her and sending "I love you" cards, I could reach out to those around me as I encountered other women who needed comfort and remind them that God is our hope and help.

Months later, after our daughter's successful surgery and recovery, I had a whole new respect for the many promises of peace made throughout Scripture. Today I strive to cling to the truth of Christ's words: "Peace I leave with you; my peace I give you. I do not give to you as the world gives. Do not let your hearts be troubled and do not be afraid" (John 14:27). I pray those dear words will become your motto as you too learn to trade anxiety for trust in the peace, goodness, and help of our loving Father.

Reflections

What do you most desire to remember about today's material?

_____

_____

Daily Exercise Prompt

Work through your Cardio TRAIN chart.

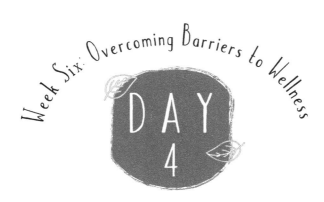

CONFRONTING SLEEP ISSUES

Closely tied to the topic of stress management is that of sleep deprivation. Most adults need between seven and eight hours of rest nightly to function at their best, but many of us get only a fraction of that. Reasons vary from having overburdened schedules, to pain, to being unable to shut out the noise of our own thoughts.

To gauge how well you are sleeping, you may want to take a short quiz from the *Sleep and Health Journal* titled "Are You Sleep Deprived?" You may find it here: sleepandhealth.com/are-you-sleep-deprived-short-quiz.

Sleep Aids

Whether your sleep issues are constant or sporadic, more tied to the process of going to sleep or more linked with staying asleep, the following helps are meant to get you on track to having a peaceful night's rest more often than not. "In peace I will lie down and sleep, for you alone, LORD, make me dwell in safety" (Psalm 4:8). Snuggle in bed at night covered with God's peace.

First, let's make sure we know the source of our rest. In Matthew 11:28 Jesus said, "Come to me, all you who are weary and burdened, and I will give you rest." All the stuff we carry can be placed confidently at the feet of our Lord. He has promised rest to those who look to Him for help and strength. Psalm 127:2 clarifies that not just the ability to rest but also sleep itself are gifts granted to us by God: "In vain you rise early and stay up late, toiling for food to eat—for he grants sleep to those he loves."

With those happy thoughts in mind, consider these further keys leading to top-quality rest.

1. Investing in a new mattress, pillow, or soft sheets facilitates nighttime comfort. Mattresses are especially important. Arya Nick Shamie, MD, associate professor of orthopedic surgery and neurosurgery, states, "The mattress needs to support your body in a neutral position, one in which your spine has nice curvature and your buttocks, heels, shoulders, and head are supported in proper alignment."[13] If you haven't replaced your mattress for several years, take your pillow to the mattress store and lie down for ten to fifteen minutes on a model or two. If you experience a significant increase in comfort compared with what you are accustomed to, it's probably time for an upgrade.

2. Creating a quality sleeping environment. The room should be dark (wear a sleep mask if necessary), cool, and cut off from the distractions of light and noise from electronics. Do not sleep in the room where you work.

3. Setting a bedtime and keeping it honors the body's natural rhythms. Ideally, we should rise at the same time daily, whether midweek or weekend.

4. Establishing a bedtime routine can train the brain to downshift, making for a less jarring transition to sleep. Consider taking a bath

---

13   Lisa Zamosky, "How to Pick Your Perfect Mattress." *WebMD: http://www.webmd.com/sleep-disorders/features/how-to-pick-your-perfect-mattress#1* (August 16, 2016).

about an hour before going to bed each night. Then prepare a cup of warm decaffeinated herbal tea such as chamomile or peppermint with a teaspoon of honey to sip during an evening devotion session. Following processes like these may help you relax.

5. Settle into bed with God on your mind. Every evening, tell the Lord good night, thanking Him for the day and placing any lingering stress in His hands one more time. Invite Him to speak to you through your dreams and to protect you from nightmares.

6. Drift off to dreamland by counting backward from 1,000, by counting your blessings, or by refusing to envision anything other than a completely blank canvas. Following steps like these can help your brain tune out anything that hinders its journey to rest.

If you have frequent sleep problems despite making such adjustments, talk to your doctor. A physician can assess you for possible sleep disorders and recommend safe and effective sleep medication. Sometimes taking a prescription sleep aid for only a few nights can reset your body's clock and encourage better rest in the future.

The Lord can set us free of fear, addiction, stress, and sleep issues. His precious help and peace are free for the taking. Will you join me in reaching out to accept His gifts?

Reflections

What point do you most hope to remember about today's material?

_____

_____

Daily Exercise Prompt

Continue working through all your TRAIN chart.

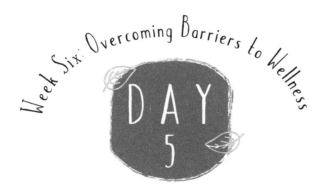

DAY 5

ABIDING IN CHRIST

I can't believe we've reached our final lesson together! I hope you feel you've grown in strength and knowledge over the last six weeks as we've discussed everything from weight management and nutrition to the various forms of exercise and common barriers to wellness. How very much I wish I could be there to hug you and celebrate alongside you! Friend, I am so proud of you for staying the course.

At the beginning of this book I shared about a beautiful and complex relationship existent between every Christ follower and our loving Creator God. I explained that we are all grafted into the Lord's family because of our association with Jesus the vine and are thus lovingly tended by God our vinedresser. I also linked the Holy Spirit to the role of a water master since He carries the things of God—love, joy, peace, patience, kindness, goodness, faithfulness, gentleness, and self-control—into our lives and helps us produce those same qualities through actions. These qualities, which I like to think of as character traits, aid us throughout our fitness and life journeys.

Today we will focus on the one fruit of the Spirit we've not yet discussed. And frankly, we must keep up the production of this particular fruit if we are to make wellness and daily dedication to serving God realties. Our final trip to the horn of plenty leads us to the trait of faithfulness.

Hebrews 11:1 defines *faith* this way: "Now faith is confidence in what we hope for and assurance about what we do not see."

"The Greek term for *faith* is *pistis,*" *The Hebrew-Greek Key Word Study Bible* explains.[14] "In the New Testament usage of faith, [the word is] frequently employed . . . to indicate trust in Jesus' ability and willingness to meet both physical and spiritual needs."[15] So *faith* is "confidence in what we hope for and assurance about what we do not see" as related to Jesus as our ultimate provider. And faith*fulness* is choosing to keep our relationship to Christ at the forefront of our thoughts and actions. It's making continual allegiance to Him the most important thing in our life.

You may recall that I chose to represent faithfulness with the picture of a pomegranate. If you've ever sliced into one of these fruits, you know they contain what can seem like an endless supply of seeds. To me this offers a fitting visual representation of how faith in God and dedication to Him should not be something in short supply. Rather, our faith and faithfulness should come in ongoing measures.

Which of the following best describes your usual level of faithfulness to pursuing Jesus?

 I'm faithful. I'm somewhat faithful. I'm hot and then cold. I'm unfaithful.

---

14   Zodhiates and Baker, *Hebrew-Greek Key Word Study Bible NIV,* 1662.

15   Ibid.

No matter how you responded to that last question, know that Jesus Christ calls us to remain *completely* committed to Him—as if we are His bride, the treasure of His heart. He tells us to abide in Him, to curl into and to trust in His love and provision no matter what may come. This involves regular Bible study, prayer, and obedience. Thus, the key to faithfulness is anchoring ourselves to Christ as our greatest passion and lifeline.

Whether your aim is to make wise wellness choices, to live morally, or to share biblical truth regularly, you cannot ignore the vital necessity of abiding in Christ. Jesus explained this well in John 15:4–9 (NASB):

> Abide in Me, and I in you. As the branch cannot bear fruit of itself unless it abides in the vine, so neither can you unless you abide in Me. I am the vine, you are the branches; he who abides in Me and I in him, he bears much fruit, for apart from Me you can do nothing. If anyone does not abide in Me, he is thrown away as a branch and dries up; and they gather them, and cast them into the fire and they are burned. If you abide in Me, and My words abide in you, ask whatever you wish, and it will be done for you. My Father is glorified by this, that you bear much fruit, and so prove to be My disciples. Just as the Father has loved Me, I have also loved you; abide in My love.

Bless you, sweet sister, for remaining faithful to our study in your pursuit of spiritual and physical wellness! I pray that you will have a lifetime of abiding in Christ, who is always faithful.

Reflections

What do you most hope to remember about today's material?

_____

_____

Daily Exercise Prompt

Work through your cardio TRAIN today. And remember—TRAINs can change and grow with you. Feel free to substitute new exercises for old ones every month or so.

Leader's Guide

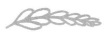

LEADER'S GUIDE
MEETING 1

Thank you for choosing to facilitate this study. Your first group meeting will serve as a get-to-know-you session in which you overview the content and invite the Lord to work in the hearts of your group members over the coming seven weeks.

Before the Session

Unless the participants are bringing their own books, get a copy of *The Strong Temple: A Woman's Guide to Developing Spiritual and Physical Health* *for each person. You and your class will be doing a brief, simple workout at your meeting, so choose a roomy gathering area, and ask everyone to wear comfortable clothing. (Don't worry if you've never led such exercises before. This guide will lead you.) Arrive early to set up your meeting place, and ask a friend to help you prepare healthful refreshments. Suggestions include water with Crystal Light options, Vitamin Water, green teas, and celery with peanut butter or Laughing Cow Cheese inside. If you'd like to play Christian music as a background for your guests' arrival time, prepare accordingly.*

Part of the first session will involve teaching the fruit of the Spirit from Galatians 5:22–23 with the goal of helping participants better understand our main verses from 1 Corinthians 3:16–17 and 6:19–20. You may either create your own signs or watch and learn from this video ahead of time to prepare: https://www.youtube.com/watch?v=FiBMSHcu4ZQ.[1] (The explanation on sign language is from 2:18 to 6:22 minutes.)

---

1   Beth Moore, "Galatians 5:22–23 with Sign Language." Posted July 11, 2013. *Living Beyond Yourself*: *https://www.youtube.com/watch?v=FiBMSHcu4ZQ* (June 22, 2016).

During the Session

1. Visit with each participant as she arrives, giving her a nametag and book at the door.

2. Enlist a helper to create a list sheet for praises and prayer requests. You may use one page for both, or you may leave several around the room.

3. Open in prayer, asking God to strengthen participants as they learn to care for their physical temples and to deepen their spiritual walks.

4. Make introductions: ask each participant to state her name and her favorite way to exercise (hiking, walking, swimming, Zumba, and so on).

5. Present "The Dash" poem. View it on the Internet at www. thedashmovie.com or https://www.facebook.com/LindaEllisAuthor/videos/273790149316398/

6. Or, read it chorally, or select a participant to read it aloud. Then discuss these questions:

   - What kind of legacy do you wish to leave?

   - Are you proud of the spiritual legacy you are building? Why or why not?

   - Are you proud of the physical legacy you are building? Explain.

   - How might having a healthier physical and spiritual temple help you create a better legacy?

7. Overview *The Strong Temple's* **content:** *Take a few minutes to skim through the Introduction and Contents with the group. Then ask, "What do you hope to gain from this study?"*

8. Share scriptures: Ask for two volunteers to read aloud. Have one read 1 Corinthians 3:16–17. The other should read 1 Corinthians

6:19–20. Say, "Our study is based on these two scriptures." Ask participants to explain how these scriptures speak to their hearts.

9. Help participants build familiarity with the fruit of the Spirit by sharing a drawing (diagram C in week 1 day 3 is an example) and by labeling individual pieces of fruit with the terms in the Galatians 5:22–23 passage or by sharing the signs available at the web address listed above. Say, "Because our bodies are temples of the Lord, we should seek to live in ways that honor Him. The fruit of the Spirit should be evident in our life."

10. Have everyone fill out the Exercise Readiness Questionnaire on page 12 to see whether any group members need to consult with their doctors before aerobically exercising.

11. Lead the group in exercise, but make allowances for anyone who forgot to wear comfy clothes and shoes or who needs to speak with a doctor first. Take participants outside and walk around your facility or up and down your street for five to ten minutes at a nice steady pace. While you walk, talk to the ladies about things for which you are grateful. (Note that when we walk, our heads should be held high. Arms should swing alternately with leg movements: right arm and left foot forward. Walkers should breathe in through the nose and out the mouth, maintaining a natural stride.)

12. End your walk with some basic stretching exercises. Refer to Appendix B, the Stretching Guide, for specific ideas and succinct directions. Each stretch should be done twice and held for ten to sixty seconds at a time. Bouncing is highly discouraged.

13. Close the session in prayer. Don't forget to refer to the praise and prayer list(s) compiled at the beginning of the session.

14. Remind participants to complete week 1's five days of content before the next group session.

15. Don't forget to send out an encouraging thank-you text or email to all participants before your next meeting.

MEETING 2

A SUMMARY OF <u>WEEK 1'S</u> READING

Before the Session

Set up the room where you are meeting with comfortable seating, paper and pens for making your praise and prayer list(s), and healthy refreshments. Consider providing tap or filtered water or Crystal Light. A variety of apples, celery (with peanut butter or Laughing Cow spread in the center), carrot sticks, and an assortment of sliced colored bell peppers make healthful snacks. You will also want to acquire one small mirror for each participant or one mirror for each table.

During the Session

1   Visit with participants as they arrive, encouraging them to add to the praise and prayer list(s) as they mingle. Thank them for coming.

2   Open in prayer: *Abba, Father, fill us with Your Holy Spirit. May we allow You the vinedresser, Jesus the vine, and the Holy Spirit to guide our choices and help us care for our precious temples both spiritually and physically.*

3   Summarize the testimony from day 1's content. Ask, "What's the difference between having a head knowledge of Christ and a heart knowledge of Him?" Discuss the importance of placing faith

in Jesus. See Appendix A should anyone have questions about accepting Christ.

4. As a group, turn through week 1's content. Encourage participants to share their thoughts and questions regarding what they read.

5. Ask participants to identify their favorite spiritual fruit and why it appeals.

6. Hand out mirrors and ask, "What do you see when you look in the mirror? What do you hope God sees when He looks at you?" Discuss what God sees: He loves us. He designed us. He has plans for us.

7. Turn to the Wellness Survey on page 43. Allow participants a few moments to respond to the survey if they have not already done so, and then ask for volunteers to share their results. Take care to encourage participants in what they are doing well and to remind them that this study will help them make positive changes as needed.

8. Lead the group in exercise. Take participants outside and walk around your facility or up and down your street for ten minutes at a steady pace. While you walk, ask participants to share ways they were able to express or witness a fruit of the Spirit this past week.

9. End your walk with the stretches covered in this week's exercise prompts: toe touches, correct hurdler's stretch, and calf and quad stretches.

10. Close the session in prayer. Don't forget to refer to the praise and prayer list(s) compiled at the beginning of the session.

11. Remind participants to complete week 2's five days of content before the next group session.

MEETING 3

A SUMMARY OF <u>WEEK 2'S</u> READING

Before the Session

Set up the room where you are meeting by providing healthful refreshments. Consider purchasing a container of Arizona Green Tea; an assortment of almonds, pecans, and walnuts; some grape tomatoes; and avocados filled with chicken or tuna salad. You will also need a tray on which the following foods are arranged artfully: carrot rounds, cross-sections of tomato, grapes, shelled walnuts, kidney beans, celery, avocadoes, eggplants, figs or pomegranates, sweet potatoes, olives, oranges, and onions. (This produce will help participants respond to the worksheet "God's Pharmacy.")

During the Session

1. Visit with participants as they arrive, encouraging them to add to the praise and prayer list(s) as they mingle. Thank them for coming.

2. Open in prayer: *Abba, Father, please allow Your Holy Spirit to transform our temples. Enable us to have the patience to make healthy choices both spiritually and physically. May we view our bodies the way You do. We are beautifully and wonderfully made. Help us reach our goals and follow our vision statements. Amen.*

3. Ask, "What does spiritual wellness involve? And what does physical wellness look like?" (See week 2 day 1 if participants need help.)

4 Ask for volunteers to explain what it means to them to know they are unique designer's originals (week 2 day 2).

5 Encourage two or three participants to share their STRONG goals with the group. Allow opportunity for the women to collect phone numbers (see page 66) to be used for accountability purposes. Remind them of the benefits of sending one another encouraging calls or texts throughout the week.

6 Turn to week 2 day 4, and focus on the formula provided there. Discuss the necessity of heart change in reaching goals.

7 Encourage participants to share their personal mission statements as related to fitness. Close that discussion by sharing your own statement.

8 Ask for and address any other questions or concerns related to the week 2 content.

9 Ask participants to turn to pages 216 and 217 while a volunteer is distributing Bibles to those who need them. Have them fill in the worksheet "God's Creation of Food," and then briefly discuss answers.

10 Have all the ladies view the tray of foods, prepared before class, for God's Pharmacy. They should look at the foods on the tray for clues as to what health benefits each fruit or veggie provides for "God's Pharmacy" and discuss. (The round cross-section of a whole carrot, for instance, should reveal the shape of a human eye.) Ask participants to complete the worksheet and then briefly discuss their answers.

11 Lead the group in exercise. Put on some lively praise and worship music. Allow participants to move in their own ways to the music. You may even set it up as a follow- the-leader experience. If so, allow each participant to lead, if she wishes to, for about thirty seconds. Try to keep moving for fifteen minutes, and have fun! End your exercising by walking for several minutes to cool down and then doing stretches from Appendix B.

12 Close the session in prayer. Don't forget to refer to the praise and prayer list(s) compiled at the beginning of the session.

13 Remind participants to complete week 3's five days of content before the next group session. Express enthusiasm over the nutritional information included there.

GOD'S CREATION OF FOOD

Grab your Bible and answer these questions about our food supply.

1 Look up Genesis 1:29–30. What did God provide humans and animals to eat in the beginning?

2 What heavenly body did He make on day 4 to support the existence of this food supply? See Genesis 1:14–19.

3 How did God describe His creations, including humans and animals, on day 6? (See Genesis 1:31.)

4 Compare the answer you gave for question 1 with Genesis 9:3, a passage in which God gave Noah instructions regarding food when he exited the ark. What had changed?

5 Read 1 Corinthians 10:31. How should foods of all types be consumed?

GOD'S PHARMACY

Match the following columns to identify ways in which the foods God created for our consumption were designed not just for nourishment but also for supportive care. The following is adapted from the article "God's Pharmacy: Interesting Facts about Fruits, Nuts, and Vegetables."[2]

Match the foods to their nutritional counterparts. Consider the way the following foods look to find clues as to their importance.

1. _____ Carrot

2. _____ Tomato

3. _____ Grape

4. _____ Walnut

5. _____ Kidney bean

6. _____ Celery

7. _____ Avocado, eggplant

8. _____ Fig/pomegranate

9. _____ Sweet potato

10. _____ Olive

11. _____ Orange

12. _____ Onion

a. supports the body's cells

b. assists in the health of ovaries

c. supports the human eye

d. looks like the blood cell

e. heals and maintains kidney function

f. increases health and function of womb

g. supports heart health

h. targets bone strength

i. helps develop transmission in brain

j. assists in breast health

k. balances the glycemic index, helping with the pancreas

l. helps lower male sterility[3]

2   "God's Pharmacy: Interesting Facts about Fruits, Nuts, and Vegetables." Posted 2016. *Top Ten Home Remedies:* http://www.top10homeremedies.com/news-facts/gods-pharmacy-interesting-facts-about-fruits-nuts-and-vegetables.html (July 12, 2016).

3   *Answers: 1-c, 2-g, 3-d, 4-i, 5-e, 6-h, 7-f, 8-l, 9-k, 10-b, 11-j, 12-a*

MEETING 4

A SUMMARY OF <u>WEEK 3'S</u> CONTENT

Before the Session

Set up your meeting place, and ask a friend to help you prepare healthful refreshments based on ideas within week 3's content. Don't forget to provide pens and paper for your prayer and praise list(s).

During the Session

1. Visit with participants as they arrive, encouraging them to add to the praise and prayer list(s) as they mingle. Thank them for coming.

2. Open in prayer: *Dear God, our vinedresser and the potter who has made us with such loving care, may every woman in this room know that she is "fearfully and wonderfully made," as Psalm 139:14 teaches. And out of that understanding, may we be good to our bodies. Lord, help us make wise choices and reach and maintain healthy BAIs and recommended weights so we may be our healthiest selves in the remaining years You provide us. May we use our precious temples to glorify You!*

3. Ask, "Why is BAI a preferred measurement over BMI alone?" (See week 3 day 2.) Discuss the necessity of having some fat, asking participants to explain fat's importance.

4   Discuss the six principles for weight management. Ask, "What changes have you made based on what you learned in this week's reading?"

5   Ask participants to share about their grocery shopping and food prep experiences this week based on tips they picked up in week 3 day 5.

6   Pass out blank postcards. Ask individuals to write down their names and addresses (e-mail) on the right side of the cards and to switch cards with the person on their left. Encourage them to write out favorite healthy recipes on the left sides of the cards when they get home. Then throughout the week they should send the recipes to one another.

7   Lead the group in exercise: Pair up and head outside for a twenty-minute walk. As you go, talk about wise nutrition choices. Don't forget to stretch before you conclude.

8   Close in prayer. Refer to the praise and prayer list(s) compiled at the beginning of the session.

9   Remind participants to complete week 4's five days of content before the next group session.

MEETING 5

A SUMMARY OF <u>WEEK 4'S</u> CONTENT

Before the Session

Set up the room where you meet. You'll need pens and paper for the prayer and praise list(s), and you may choose to bring in appropriate music for this week's exercise segment. Enlist the help of a friend in providing the participants with green tea and in preparing the following dishes. (Or you may want to substitute some of your own healthy recipes.)

TOSSED GREEN SALAD

Ingredients

1 head of green-tip lettuce, 1 bag of spring mix, 1 bag of fresh spinach
Add any healthy ingredients talked about last week—bright veggies, healthy nuts
1 tablespoon of olive oil
1 lemon

Preparation

Toss all the first ingredients in a bowl.
Add the olive oil, and squeeze the lemon right before serving.

DANETTE'S HEALTHY COOKIE DOUGH BALLS

Nutritionist, personal trainer, and figure competitor Danette May has come up with tasty and healthy recipes for her whole family to enjoy. Try her cookie dough balls.

Nutritional Information
2 balls = 3 oz. protein, 1 tbsp. fat, 1/4 cup carbs
Makes approximately 25 balls
Preparation time: 7 minutes

Ingredients
1 cup almond butter or natural peanut butter (or try both mixed half and half) 1/4 cup honey (raw, if you can find it) 3 cups dry oatmeal (Pulverize dry oats in a blender or coffee grinder first, which helps form a cookie dough texture in the final balls. I use steel-cut oatmeal.)
2–3 scoops vanilla or chocolate whey protein1/3 cup water

Optional: For added flavor, you can add 1/2 cup of coconut or dark chocolate chips or cacao nibs (70% or higher chocolate chips for less sugar).[4]

Preparation
Mix ingredients together in a bowl, and then roll into one-inch balls. Eat a couple right away, or freeze for an on-the-go treat anytime.

During the Session

1   Visit with participants as they arrive, encouraging them to add to the praise and prayer list(s) as they mingle. Thank them for coming.

2   Open in prayer: *Abba, Father, please help us have healthy, kind hearts. Please forgive us for our sins, and equip us to care for our spiritual and physical hearts in ways that glorify You. Amen.*

---

4   Danette May, "7-Minute Healthy Cookie Dough Balls." *Okuma Nutritionals*: http://www. wulongforlife.com/7-minute-healthy-cookie-dough-balls/ (September 5, 2016).

3. Ask participants to turn to week 4 day 1. Encourage them to share what they learned about the heart's spiritual importance. Ask, "Who identified more with Eliab? With David? What can we do to be more like David in the matter of having a clean heart?"

4. Summarize TRAIN (week 4 day 2), and ask for a volunteer to share her complete cardio-TRAIN plan to date. Reiterate that TRAIN can and will be modified and expanded in the weeks ahead.

5. Ask, "Which Bible verses can help us to persevere in the pursuit of wellness? In spiritual matters?"

6. Encourage participants to share their favorite ways to stay active that do not feel like traditional exercise. Start with a list of your own.

7. Acknowledge that heart problems will continue to plague humanity until the Lord's return: disease is a part of the curse of sin. Good things, however, can come out of even health struggles. Read aloud the testimony below, and then ask the related question that follows.

> My mother was a smoker for over thirty years, ate whatever she wanted, and ended up having a heart attack in 1999 that almost took her life. The doctors said that the combination of smoking and unhealthy foods had clogged her arteries, and they recommended she have triple bypass surgery. It would require them to harvest veins in her leg and then transplant them into her heart to improve her circulation. In the two months following that procedure, Mom almost died twice.
>
> This was a terrible time for our family, but my brother—seeing our mother go through this horrible sickness—decided to give up smoking as a result. My family, friends, and pastor, who prayed so faithfully for Mom during her illness, got to see God work in an amazing way. My mother lived twelve years beyond her heart struggle, though doctors expected

she'd not survive far past it. I thank God for meeting us and working even in our pain. —J.J.

8   Ask, "What does this testimony suggest about the Lord? Do you have a similar testimony about a way God showed Himself faithful or brought good out of a heart-related struggle? If so, please share it."

9   On the back of the prayer and praise list, work with participants to compile a record of the cardio exercises they have been working on this week. With the goal of working out today for a total of twenty-five minutes, incorporate as many of those exercises as possible into your group exercise time. Keep it fun, and don't forget to cool down with some stretches.

10   Close in prayer.

11   Assign week 5's content. It should be completed prior to your next group session.

MEETING 6

A SUMMARY OF <u>WEEK 5'S</u> CONTENT

Before the Session

If you'd like to switch things up this week and have a contact who is willing to volunteer, enlist the help of a personal trainer to close out this group session in a no-equipment-needed workout. Then set up the room where you are meeting. Enlist a friend's help in preparing refreshments. The goal is to reward hard-working participants with this relaxing meal:

- Finger sandwiches of Orowheat® whole grain and flax bread, lean turkey, low-fat mayo, and lettuce

- Fruit salad made with dark berries

- Chamomile, lemon balm, and/or peppermint hot (cold) tea with a teaspoon of honey per eight-ounce cup[5]

During the Session

1   Visit with participants as they arrive, encouraging them to add to the praise and prayer list(s) as they mingle. Thank them for coming.

2   Open in prayer: *Dear Father, we rejoice that You have provided us this opportunity to learn how to make wise choices for the benefit of our*

---

5   Note that turkey contains tryptophan, an amino acid that induces sleep. Dark-colored berries contain antioxidants that help prevent and fight cancer. The teas are believed to be stress-alleviating and can also help induce a good night's rest.

precious temples. Lord, please help us as we train our bodies and our hearts to be the best they can be for Your glory. We praise You that a day is coming when we will see You face to face and will be given bodies gloriously made new. In Jesus's name. Amen.

} Turn to week 5 day 1, and ask participants to share their thoughts on that day's content. Then read this story aloud:

> Author Kathryn Baker tells of her grandmother, who loved Psalm 103:2-5. It says, "Praise the LORD, O my soul, and forget not all his benefits—who forgives all your sins and heals all your diseases, who redeems your life from the pit and crowns you with love and compassion, who satisfies your desires with good things so that your youth is renewed like the eagle's." Even today this passage reminds Kathryn that God is our trustworthy healer—even when it may seem that He is inactive.

> When her friend Robin died in middle school, Kathryn was confused as to why God had not answered prayers requesting that He heal her friend of leukemia. To this Kathryn's grandmother responded with her knowledge of God's Word. 'Honey,' she said, 'God heals in three ways. The first is instantaneous. We pray and God answers immediately with a miracle—whether He uses medicine or something that defies explanation. The second way God heals is over time. You pray, family and friends pray, and a person is healed either through natural processes, doctor intervention, or miracle. But the third way is actually the best way because it's the only one that lasts. Sometimes God heals by calling us home. In heaven we'll get bodies restored to the perfection He always intended. I can't think of any better way to be healed than that.

4   Ask participants to respond to the story. (Be aware that the third type of healing is a promise made only to those who belong to Jesus and are called home in God's timing.)

5   Discuss the benefits of gaining muscle tone, as presented in week 5 day 2.

6   Ask, "What did you learn about strength training this week that surprised you or encouraged you to incorporate it into your routine?"

7   Discuss the additions made to TRAIN chart this week. Encourage participants to stay the course.

8   Request that participants share insights they gained in week 5 day 5. Ask, "Who do you know that lives out the kind of spiritual flexibility and readiness to share the gospel presented in this week's chapter? How can you become more like that?"

9   Remind participants that next week's session is the last. Encourage them to prepare healthful recipes for the next session that can be shared in a group potluck. Individuals will also need to bring a list of their favorite exercises: one cardio, one strength building, and one stretch (each on a separate note card).

10   Lead the group in thirty minutes of exercise, either using your own TRAIN routine or allowing a personal trainer to take everyone through a simple workout.

11   Close in prayer, taking care to incorporate requests and praises on this week's list.

MEETING 7

A SUMMARY OF <u>WEEK 6'S</u> CONTENT

Before the Session

Set up the room where you are meeting, and ready a prayer and praise list. Request the help of a volunteer to prepare for this session's potluck meal and to place foods as they arrive.

During the Session

1. Welcome participants as they arrive, collecting their lists of exercises assigned at the close of last week's meeting (one cardio, one strength-train, and one stretch).

2. Open in prayer: *Dear Abba, Father, we thank You for all we've learned over the course of this study. Please bless our time together, and continue to enable us to reflect and express Your fruit of the Spirit and to have a deeper growing relationship with You. May all that we've studied continue to encourage us to make wise wellness choices that will improve and strengthen the temples You've created. May we use them to glorify You daily and to share the gospel faithfully. Help us to abide in You. Amen.*

3. Encourage participants to fill their plates with the healthful refreshment options they provided and to add to the prayer and praise list(s) as needed.

4. Turn to week 6. Ask for a volunteer to read aloud Psalm 139:16. Discuss the verse in relation to overcoming a fear of cancer and health concerns in general. Ask, "What does this verse tell us about God's interest in our lives?"

5. Ask, "What did you take away from reading Philippians 4:4–9?"

6. Share reflections and favorite verses from week 6 day 2.

7. Take turns sharing your multi-step, anti-stress prescriptions from week 6 day 3. Then if time allows, ask participants to share their own methods for falling asleep and staying asleep.

8. Ask, "What has been most helpful to you regarding your understanding of either the fruit of the Spirit or physical temple care during our study?"

9. Select from among the favorite exercises participants submitted at the start of class to assemble a workout routine of approximately thirty minutes. If you are unsure as to how to do a particular exercise, ask the individual who submitted it to demonstrate. Limit each exercise to one set of three reps. Hold each stretch for ten to sixty seconds.

10. Thank participants for coming, encourage them to continue to TRAIN—alternating in new exercises when things start to feel stale—and then close in prayer.

APPENDIX A

How to Know You Are a Born-Again Christian

Some people wander through life uncertain of where they will spend eternity. The Bible is clear that there are only two end destinations: heaven and hell. Entry into the former is something about which we can be certain. In 1 John 5:13 the beloved disciple said, "I write these things to you who believe in the name of the Son of God [that's Jesus!] *so that you may know that you have eternal life*" *(emphasis mine).*

If you can't confidently say you are a born-again Christian, ask yourself these questions:

1   **Do I recognize that I am a sinner, a person who commits wrongs against God?**
    The Bible says, "All have sinned and fall short of the glory of God" (Romans 3:23), and everything from lying to having murderous thoughts to just plain failing to do the right thing counts as sin. Those who truly belong to Jesus Christ know they are hopelessly destined to displease God without His help.

2   **Do I believe God sacrificed His Son, Jesus, to pay the death penalty that I, in my sins, deserve? And do I also affirm that God raised Jesus from the dead?**
    Divine Jesus came to earth in human form so He could live a sinless life and act as a substitutionary sacrifice, appeasing God's wrath against all who would come to Him in faith. He also rose three days after His crucifixion to demonstrate His power over death and to assure His followers that they too would receive life beyond the

grave. This is the truth behind John 3:16–17: "For God so loved the world that he gave his one and only Son, that whoever believes in him shall not perish but have eternal life. For God did not send his Son into the world to condemn the world, but to save the world through him."

) **Do I confidently confess with my mouth that Jesus died for me?**
Romans 10:9 says, "If you declare with your mouth, 'Jesus is Lord,' and believe in your heart that God raised him from the dead, you will be saved [from the penalty your sins deserve and from the curse of death]."

If you answered yes to all the above questions, you can take comfort in Christ's words: "Very truly I tell you, the one who believes has eternal life" (John 6:47). Praise be to the Lord that you are a saved daughter of the King!

If you answered no, be assured that God loves you dearly. If you'll approach Him through faith in His Son, He will call you His own this very day. (Please see my own prayer to accept Him on page 20.)

APPENDIX B

Stretching Guide

AMERICAN COLLEGE OF SPORTS MEDICINE'S
MOST RECENT GUIDELINES

"Stretching should be done at least 2 to 3 days a week; however, greater gains will be attained if done daily. It involves holding a body part stationary for 30 to 60 seconds for older persons, 10 to 30 seconds for most adults." [6] Static stretching refers to elongating or bending a warm muscle or group of warm muscles to lengthen that muscle so it will become more flexible, less prone to stiffness.

Before engaging in any of the stretching suggestions below, warm your muscles for three to five minutes by running in place, doing jumping jacks, or through performing any of the cardio suggestions made in this study. As you begin stretching, remember not to bounce. While you should extend a muscle to the point of tightness, you should not push yourself to the point of discomfort. Always take care to breathe steadily.

Ideally, you should perform one set of three to five reps for each stretch. A "set" is made up of a fixed number of repetitions. A "rep" is the number of times a muscle or group of muscles is worked within a set. One set of toe touches may have seven reps, ending with a rest.

STRETCHES

---

6   Barber et al. "ACSM's Flexibility Training Exercise Design Guidelines," by the American College of Sports Medicine. 2011. https://www.anatomytrains.com/wp-content/uploads/manual/acsm.docx (November 5, 2016).

Below are basic directions for completing common stretches. They have been divided according to which region of the body they chiefly address. If you feel uncertain about how to do a stretch based on the information given, please skip it or look online for more information.

Please note that you will complete one set of two to four reps for each exercise. (Beginners need do only one set of two reps.) Each stretch should be held at the point of mild discomfort—not pain—for ten to sixty seconds.

FLOOR STRETCHES

I. LOWER BODY STRETCHES

a. Toe touches

Step 1: *Sit on the floor, and straighten your back with your legs in front of you so your body is in the shape of an L. Keep your feet and legs together.*

Step 2: *Place your hands on your knees and bend forward slowly, reaching toward your toes. Remember to keep your legs as straight as possible.*

Step 3: *Exhale as you reach. When you feel you cannot safely stretch further, hold it and then gently relax back into an upright position, rest, and repeat.*

b. Hurdler's stretch

Step 1: *Sit on the floor, and straighten your right leg at a 45-degree angle to your right side. Bend your left knee, and rest your left heel against your groin.*

Step 2: *Laying your hands one on top of the other, stretch your upper body toward the outstretched toe and hold before resting.*

Step 3: *Repeat the exercise for the opposite side of your body.*

c. Butterfly stretch

Step 1: *Sit on the floor with your back straight. Bring the soles of your shoes together in front of your body so your legs are in two V shapes.*

Step 2: *Pull your feet as close to your groin area as possible, cupping your hands around your toes to hold the position.*

Step 3: *Release your feet, and use the palms of your hands to gently push your knees toward the floor. Hold.*

II. CORE/MID-SECTION

a. Cat and cow stretch

Step 1: *Get down on all fours, positioning your hands under your shoulders and your knees under your hips. Your palms and the tops of your feet should be flat on the floor.*

Step 2: *Look at your thighs, pressing your hands into the floor as you push your spine toward the ceiling in an arch shape. This is the "cat" portion of the stretch. Hold.*

Step 3: *Slowly bring your face upward until you are looking directly in front of you. As you do, gently lower your back until it makes a slight U shape. Shoulders and tailbone should be raised above the middle of the back. This is the "cow" portion of the stretch. Hold.*

b. Turtle stretch

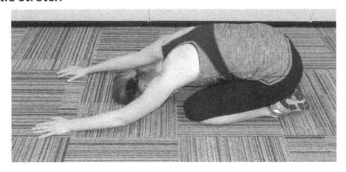

Turtle Stretch

233

Step 1: *Kneel so you are sitting on your heels.*

Step 2: *Gently collapse forward to rest your chest on your thighs, forming a loose ball shape with your body. Your forehead should touch the floor.*

Step 3: *Keep your arms out in front of your body, allowing your palms to rest on the floor. Hold.*

III. UPPER BODY

a. Neck stretches

Step 1: *Sit on the floor with legs crisscrossed in front of you, making the shape of an M. Rest your hands in your lap. Sit up straight, and then gently roll your shoulders back and drop them into a comfortable position. Face forward.*

Step 2: *With slow and deliberate movements, drop your forehead toward your chest, hold, and then raise and lean your head back toward your spine and hold. This is one rep.*

Step 3: *Remaining in the same basic position, lean your head so your right ear is heading downward toward your right shoulder and hold. Raise your head back to normal position. Then lean your left ear toward your left shoulder and hold. This is one rep.*

Step 4: *Remaining in the same basic position, gently turn your neck to the left and hold, and then to the right and hold. This is one rep.*

b. Scapula stretch

Step 1: *Sit tall on the floor with your legs crisscrossed in front of you.*

Step 2: *Extend both arms up, fingers pointing to the sky.*

Step 3: *Keep your elbows pointing upward as you drop your hands behind your head to touch your back. Hold.*

STANDING AND SITTING STRETCHES

I. LOWER BODY

a. Calf stretch for both legs

Step 1: *Face a wall and stand about an arm's length away from it. Your feet should be shoulder-width apart, feet flat on the floor and toes pointing toward the wall, as if you were going to perform a standing wall push-up. Take one or two steps back from the wall and lean forward.*

Step 2: *Gently bend your elbows, remaining aware of the stretching sensation you should feel in your calves. If you are not getting enough resistance, move your feet back farther or bend your arms until your forehead is closer to the wall. Hold.*

b. Calf stretch for individual legs

Step 1: *Follow the directions given under step 1 of the calf stretch for both legs.*

Step 2: *This time, move one leg toward the wall, keeping the back leg straight and the toe pointed forward. Press heel into the floor.*

Step 3: *Lean into the wall until you feel the stretch. Hold.*

Step 4: *Switch legs and repeat.*

c. Calf stretch with toe touch

Step 1: *Follow the directions given under step 1 of the calf stretch for both legs.*

Step 2: *This time, extend one leg forward, placing that foot against the baseboard as you keep the other leg extended behind you with the ball of your foot and heel on the floor.*

Step 3: *As you lean into the wall, feel for the stretch. Hold. Alternate feet.*

d. Quad stretch

Step 1: *Stand up straight with your left hand against the wall for balance. Bend your right foot back toward your buttocks. Hold onto your right toe with your right hand. The right knee should be pointing to the ground, left knee slightly bent. Keep your knees close together.*

Step 2: *Pull your foot up and back from your body. Hold.*

Step 3: *Alternate sides and repeat.*

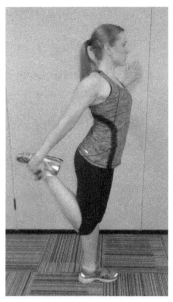

Quad stretch

e. Lunge stretch

Step 1: *Stand up straight with your right side against the edge of a couch or immoveable object. Then slowly lower your right side to the couch, straightening your left leg out behind you as in the photo.*

Step 2: *Push the ball of your left foot into the ground, and push your left hip forward to feel the stretch. Hold.*

Step 3: *Alternate sides, and repeat steps.*

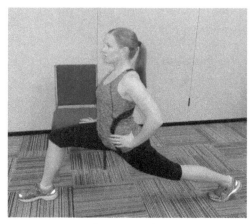

Lunge stretch

f. Hamstring stretch (hinge hips)

Step 1: *Stand tall with your hands on your hips and shoulders rolled back. Place your feet shoulder-width apart with your knees slightly bent. Throughout this exercise, think of each hip as if it were a hinge.*

Step 2: *Keeping your back straight, gradually bend at the hip area to lower your upper body toward your knees. Keep your hands on your hips to begin. Slowly lower your hands toward the ground.*

Step 3: *Feel for the stretch in your calves, quads, and/or hamstrings, depending on your specific flexibility. Hold.*

g. Newspaper stretch

Step 1: *Sit up straight in a chair with your feet on the floor.*

Step 2: *Place your right ankle on top of your left knee with your right ankle flexed. Hold your right toe with your left hand and place your right hand on your knee.*

Step 3: *Lean forward as you pull your right toe with your left hand, and push gently with your right hand on your right knee until you feel the stretch in your top leg. Hold.*

Step 4: *Alternate legs.*

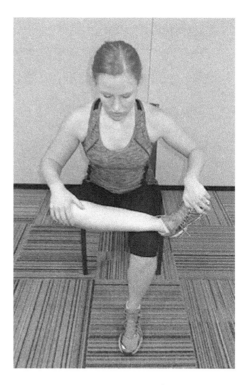

Newspaper stretch

237

IV. CORE OR MID-SECTION STRETCHES

a. Standing side stretch

Step 1: *Stand tall, with feet a little wider than shoulder-width apart. Place you left hand on your left hip with your right arm extended above your head and reaching to the left.*

Step 2: *Lean to your left as your right arm reaches to the left. Hold.*

Step 3: *Alternate arms.*

b. Press forward

Step 1: *Stand tall with knees slightly bent and arms held out in front of you parallel to the ground, the backs of your hands facing you. Interlock your fingers, and keep your palms pressing away from you.*

Step 2: *Tuck your chin to your chest.*

Step 3: *Arch and push your spine backward. Hold.*

c. Shoulder press

Step 1: *Stand tall with knees slightly bent. Keep your arms behind you, your hands interlocked.*

Step 2: *Roll your shoulders back.*

Step 3: *Push your chest forward, and slowly raise your arms. Hold.*

d. Back lean

Step 1: *Keeping your hands on your hips and your feet shoulder-width apart, knees slightly bent, face the wall in front of you.*

Step 2: *Lean back until you feel a stretch in your back. Hold.*

e. Chair stretch

Step 1: *Sit up straight in a chair with your feet on the floor. Keep your arms by your side or crisscrossed at your chest.*

Step 2: *Slowly lower your head and upper body toward your knees one vertebra at a time. Hold each position for a second.*

Step 3: *Slowly roll your back into an upright position (using your stomach muscles to perform this move).*

V. UPPER BODY STRETCHES

a. Shoulder-and-arm stretch

Step 1: *Stand tall with feet shoulder-width apart, knees slightly bent. Keep your frame facing forward throughout this stretch.*

Step 2: *Take your right arm across your chest to the left side of your body. Your right arm should remain parallel to the floor.*

Step 3: *Your left hand should hold onto your right arm between the elbow and shoulder. Hold.*

Step 4: *Switch arms.*

b. Tricep stretch

Step 1: *Stand tall with feet shoulder-width apart, knees slightly bent. Keep your frame facing forward throughout this stretch.*

Step 2: *Raise your right arm to the ceiling.*

Step 3: *Drop your right hand behind your back with your right elbow still facing the ceiling.*

Step 4: *Hold your right elbow with your left hand, and push gently down and toward your back as you exhale. Hold.*

Step 5: *Switch arms and hands.*

ABOUT THE AUTHOR

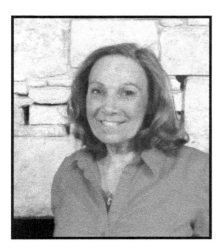

Kathryn Baker was awakened most mornings of her young life by roosters crowing, cows mooing, horses neighing, chickens clucking, dogs barking, and cats meowing. She is a native-born Texan who was raised on a working farm and ranch in central Texas. Early summers found all the family harvesting crops for livestock and vegetables that could be canned and frozen for household meals throughout the year. During warmer weather the family enjoyed playing, swimming, and skiing in the San Marcos River. Fishing and hunting were also big parts of their outdoor activities.

Kathryn was blessed early in life to be around strong Christian leaders and followers of Jesus Christ, though for many years her relationship with Him was one of head knowledge rather than faith. Nonetheless, she attended a Christian church and Sunday school as a youngster and young adult. Then after marriage she accepted Jesus as Lord and went on to raise her kids to love Him.

Her degrees are from the University of Houston. She holds a bachelor of education degree in health and physical education and a master of education degree in sports performance. Most of her time teaching was spent in Houston at The Kinkaid School. There she taught physical education for lower-school students and coached middle- and upper-school sports. A move to Bedford, Texas, in 2002 found her working on another degree at the University of Texas at Arlington, where she specialized in reading. She then began teaching that subject to kindergartners. Later, following another move, she became the assistant coach for the women's volleyball team at LeTourneau University. In the summer of 2005 she began teaching kinesiology classes to adults in LeTourneau's education department. She continues there to this day.

Kathryn and her husband are deeply involved in their church in Longview, Texas. They are active on several committees and love praying over, traveling with, and participating in mission groups. Through penning this study and teaching it in person as given the opportunity, she endeavors to demonstrate her church's mission statement: "People leading all people into a life-changing, ever-growing relationship with Jesus Christ."

CPSIA information can be obtained
at www.ICGtesting.com
Printed in the USA
BVHW031149140219
540290BV00001B/52/P